Clinical Approach to
Acne Vulgaris

Clinical Approach to
Acne Vulgaris

Kabir Sardana

MD DNB MNAMS

Professor
Department of Dermatology and
Nodal Officer STD
(Regional STD Centre)
Maulana Azad Medical College
and Lok Nayak Hospital
New Delhi

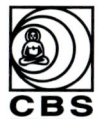

CBS

CBS Publishers & Distributors Pvt Ltd

New Delhi • Bengaluru • Chennai • Kochi • Kolkata • Mumbai • Pune
Hyderabad • Nagpur • Patna • Vijayawada

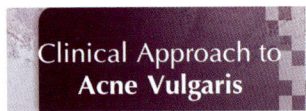

ISBN: 978-81-239-2835-7

Copyright © Author and Publisher

First Edition: 2015

Published by Satish Kumar Jain and produced by Varun Jain for

CBS Publishers & Distributors Pvt Ltd

4819/XI Prahlad Street, 24 Ansari Road, Daryaganj, New Delhi 110 002, India.
Ph: 23289259, 23266861, 23266867   Website: www.cbspd.com
Fax: 011-23243014   e-mail: delhi@cbspd.com; cbspubs@airtelmail.in.
Corporate Office: 204 FIE, Industrial Area, Patparganj, Delhi 110 092
Ph: 4934 4934   Fax: 4934 4935   e-mail: publishing@cbspd.com; publicity@cbspd.com

Branches

* **Bengaluru:** Seema House 2975, 17th Cross, K.R. Road,
  Banasankari 2nd Stage, Bengaluru 560 070, Karnataka
  Ph: +91-80-26771678/79   Fax: +91-80-26771680   e-mail: bangalore@cbspd.com
* **Chennai:** 7, Subbaraya Street, Shenoy Nagar, Chennai 600 030, Tamil Nadu
  Ph: +91-44-26260666, 26208620   Fax: +91-44-42032115   e-mail: chennai@cbspd.com
* **Kochi:** Ashana House, No. 39/1904, AM Thomas Road, Valanjambalam,
  Eranakulam 682 018, Kochi Kerala
  Ph: +91-484-4059061-65   Fax: +91-484-4059065   e-mail: kochi@cbspd.com
* **Kolkata:** 6/B, Ground Floor, Rameswar Shaw Road, Kolkata-700 014, West Bengal
  Ph: +91-33-22891126, +91-33-22891127, +91-33-22891128   e-mail: kolkata@cbspd.com
* **Mumbai:** 83-C, Dr E Moses Road, Worli, Mumbai-400018, Maharashtra
  Ph: +91-22-24902340/41   Fax: +91-22-24902342   e-mail: mumbai@cbspd.com
* **Pune:** Bhuruk Prestige, Sr. No. 52/12/2+1+3/2 Narhe, Haveli
  (Near Katraj-Dehu Road Bypass), Pune 411 041, Maharashtra
  Ph: +91-20-64704058/59, 32392277   Fax: +91-20-24300160   e-mail: pune@cbspd.com

Representatives

* **Hyderabad** 0-9885175004 * **Nagpur** 0-9021734563
* **Patna**   0-9334159340 * **Vijayawada** 0-9000660880

Printed at: HT Media Ltd., Noida, UP

Why does one get married? It is because we need a witness to our lives. There are a billion people on the planet ... . I mean, what does any one's life really mean to anyone? The good things, the bad things, the terrible things, the mundane things ... all of it, all of the time, every day... . "Your life will not go unwitnessed because I will be your witness'. That "I" is my wife, Dr Supriya, a companion and colleague, who handles everything, so that I can partake of my professional pursuits. A big thanks to you!

to
my daughter, Zoya,
who may not know, like most children,
how much we value them;

and

my parents, well wishers and fellow dermatologists

Contributors

Soumya Agarwal MD DNB (Dermatology)
Senior Resident
Lady Hardinge Medical College
Delhi

Shilpa Garg DNB (Dermatology and Venereology)
Assistant Professor
Department of Dermatology
Army College of Medical Sciences, Base Hospital
Delhi Cantt

Taru Garg MD (Dermatology)
Professor
Lady Hardinge Medical College
Delhi

Sangita Ghosh MBBS DDVL (JIPMER)
Consultant Dermatologist
Kolkata

Syeda Tanvira Habib MD
Senior Resident
VM Medical College and Safdarjung Hospital
New Delhi

Niti Khunger MD DDV DNB
Professor and Consultant Dermatologist
VM Medical College and Safdarjung Hospital
New Delhi

Anjali Madan MD
Senior Resident
Dermatology
Maulana Azad Medical College and Lok Nayak Hospital
Delhi

Abhay M Martin DVD MD DNB FIMSA
Senior Consultant Dermatologist
Division of Dermatology
Baby Memorial Hospital
Calicut

Amita Mhatre
Resident, Department of Dermatology
D.Y. Patil Hospital and School of Medicine
Nerul, Navi Mumbai

Isha Narang MBBS
Dermatology (PG 2nd Year)
Maulana Azad Medical College and Lok Nayak Hospital
Delhi

Varadraj Pai MD
Assistant Professor
Goa Medical College

Sharmila Patil
Professor and Head of Dermatology Department
D.Y.Patil Hospital and School of Medicine
Nerul, Navi Mumbai

Kabir Sardana MD DNB MNAMS
Professor
Department of Dermatology and Nodal Officer STD
(Regional STD Centre)
Maulana Azad Medical College and
Lok Nayak Hospital
New Delhi

Preface

There is a little doubt that acne is the commonest skin disorder. Sadly even amongst specialists it is the most mismanaged. A large number of persistent acne patients are acne cosmetica cases and the culprits are moisturizers, sunscreens and fairness creams. I have seen numerous cases of females with such acne. In fact the spate of beauty advertisements is a reason for the acne flares in India with the beauty clinics adding to the mess. We have, in addition, numerous home remedies and so-called safe herbal and ayurvedic products that add to the problem. Most of these target the "infection" by *P. acnes*, which is a commensal and is not the most important thing in acne.

As most patients visit the practitioner, this book is written for them. Even though dermatologists, primary care doctors, and pediatricians see these patients every day in practice, very few can appreciate the risk of physical scarring and negative psychosocial impact this disease carries. Improving the skin can improve self-confidence, interpersonal relationships, and performance in school or at work place. My interest in acne emanates on a thesis that I did in medical college on the psychological impact of acne. Now I am on the other end researching on *P. acnes* and resistance in India

This book will help to provide a broad overview of acne vulgaris itself as well as the conditions that manifest with acneiform eruptions in the skin. A targeted approach to its management encompasses the various scenarios that one may face. At the end a few points that I wish to highlight.

- Do not use steroids on the face …. all the brands ending with – ate.

- Do not use Azithromycin in acne as there are simpler and cheaper molecules available, using a class of drug that is used for other medical disorders is a crime as we have created a resistance problem of massive proportions.

- Sunscreens do not help in acne and most of them have the wrong base, thus can cause acne. No one gets fairer with sunscreens also I assure you!

- When in doubt refer, it is always honorable to refer than to mess up, specially the face.

Kabir Sardana

Contents

What and Why of Acne Vulgaris

Acne is a disorder of the pilosebaceous unit seen exclusively in humans. It affects teenagers mainly and adults occasionally. It is due to the combined effect of hormonal, inflammatory, infective and immune components.

Traditionally 4 factors have been recognised to produce acne—androgen, sebum, *Propionibacterium acnes* and abnormal keratinisation. Three other pathogenetic factors have recently attracted attention—the innate immune system with local inflammatory responses, the role of genetic factors and the influence of diet in acne (Fig. 1.1).

ROLE OF ANDROGENS

Acne has been considered an androgen sensitive disease. Androgens are produced by the gonads, adrenal gland as well as locally within

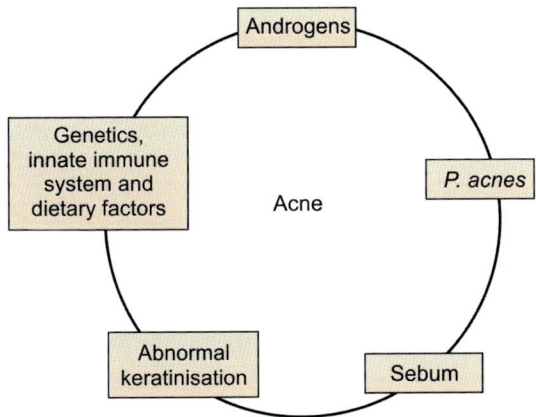

Fig. 1.1: An interplay of factors are involved in the pathogenesis of acne vulgaris

the sebaceous gland. Androgens from the adrenal and gonads are converted to testosterone and dihydrotestosterone (DHT) in the skin via 5-alpha reductase enzyme (type 1).

The fact that androgens are key determinants of acne pathophysiology is proved by several clinical and laboratory evidences.

Physiologic and Biochemical Evidences

- The sebaceous gland is under the influence of androgens for its growth and differentiation.
- Sebum production is directly influenced by androgen production.
- There is high androgen receptor density and 5-alpha reductase activity in acne prone skin.
- Blockage of enzymes of androgen synthesis or receptors can regulate sebum production.

Clinical Evidences Include

- Onset of acne occurs in puberty which coincides with a spurt in levels of androgens.
- Neonatal acne is thought to be due to the influence of maternal androgens.
- Acne is a presentation of diseases of the ovary like polycystic ovary syndrome, hormone secreting tumours, etc.
- Acne may be a presentation of adrenal diseases like congenital adrenal hyperplasia or adrenal tumours.
- Acne is absent in castrated males and patients with androgen insensitivity syndromes (lack of functional androgen receptors).

Androgens are also known to stimulate keratinocyte differentiation through growth factors and IL-1α which inturn induce hyperkeratinisation in the ductal epithelium and infundibular regions. This inturn leads to comedogenesis. These comedones are the basic hallmark of acne vulgaris.

ROLE OF SEBUM

Sebum is secreted by the sebaceous gland by holocrine secretion (extrusion of cell along with its secretion) and is composed of squalene, triglycerides, phospholipids, cholesterol and cholesterol esters and wax esters. *P. acnes* produce lipases that break down triglycerides and form mono and diglycerides and free fatty acids.

The genesis of acne is dependent on both the quantum of secretion of sebum (regulated by multiple factors mentioned below) as well as the composition of the lipids in the sebum (Fig. 1.2).

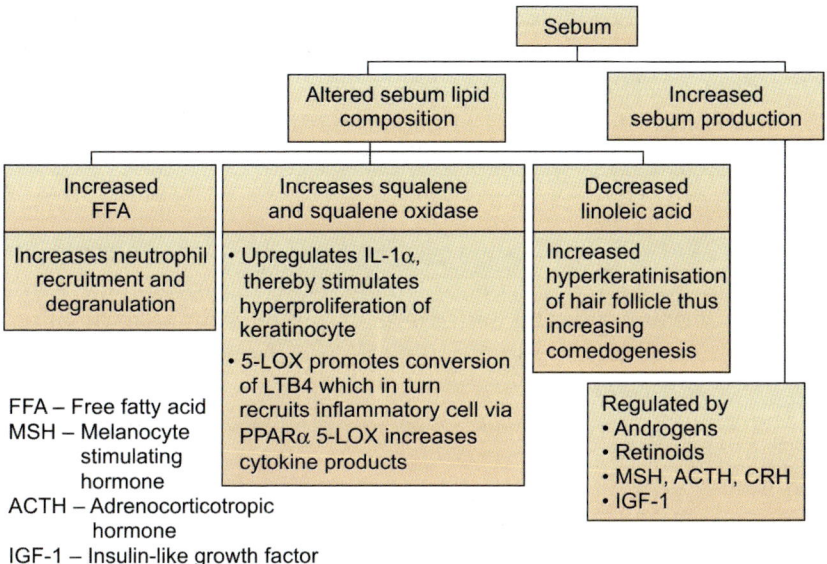

Fig. 1.2: Sebum is an essential component of acne pathogenesis: Both quantum of sebum production and lipid composition of sebum contribute to the pathogenesis

The regulation of sebum secretion is multifactorial. The key factors are discussed below:

a. *Androgens***:** Androgens stimulate sebocyte proliferation, growth and sebum production. This is achieved through androgen receptors that are present on the basal layer of the sebaceous glands.

b. *Retinoids***:** Retinoids like isotretinoin and 1-cis retinoic acid cause sebaceous gland shrinkage and inhibit sebum secretion. This is mediated through retinoid receptors and PPAR receptors.

c. *MSH, ACTH, CRH***:** Receptors for MSH (melanocyte stimulating hormone), ACTH (adrenocorticotropic hormone) and CRH (corticotropin releasing hormone) are expressed on the sebaceous glands. CRH is released in response to physiologic stress and is known to increase sebum lipid production in sebocytes *in vitro* studies.

d. *IGF-1***:** Insulin like growth factor is a physiologic element which is known to be highly expressed in insulin resistance syndromes, polycystic ovary syndrome and metabolic syndrome and correlates with the higher incidence of acne in these diseases. Dietary influences that increase acne are also postulated to be mediated through the IGF-1 pathway.

Altered Lipid Composition in Sebum

Increased sebum secretion alone is not sufficient for acne pathogenesis. Alterations in sebum composition have a major role to play in this. The role of sebum that leads up to acne formation is summarised in Fig. 1.2.

ROLE OF *P. ACNES*

Propionibacterium acnes is a normal commensal in the pilosebaceous unit found in nearly 100% of adults. *P. acnes* concentration increases during puberty in parallel with the secretion of sebum, increases up to the age of 25 and then remains constant through middle age and decreases after the age of 70.

The role of *P. acnes* in the initiation of comedogenesis or in the inflammatory processes involved has been a matter of debate. What is available as support for this is only circumstantial evidence; a favourable microenvironment leads to increased colonisation and this may in turn promote the comedogenesis. *P. acnes* can intensify the inflammatory process but is dispensable for its initiation.

P. acnes has been known to influence comedogenesis at multiple levels (Fig. 1.3).

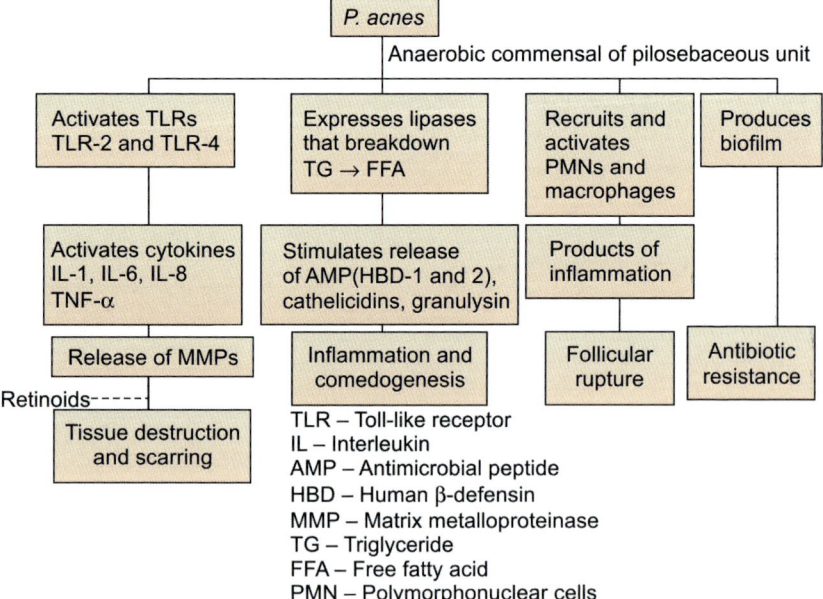

Fig. 1.3: *P. acnes* is an anaerobic commensal in the pilosebaceous unit and is considered an important trigger of comedogenesis

1. It expresses lipases that breakdown triglycerides into free fatty acids. These fatty acids stimulate the release of antimicrobial peptides (AMP) which in turn promote inflammation and comedogenesis.
2. It activates the release of Toll-like receptors,TLR-2 and TLR-4. TLR-2 mediated cytokines (IL-1, IL-6, IL-8 and TNF-α) activate the release of matrix metalloproteinases which cause tissue destruction and scar formation.
   The role of retinoids like isotretinoin and tretinoin is that it inhibits MMP induced damage, thus preventing scar formation.
3. It causes differentiation, recruitment and activation of neutrophils and macrophages in the pilosebaceous unit. Products of inflammation released from these cells are responsible for sustaining inflammation and causing follicular rupture.
4. TLRs activate the expression of antimicrobial peptides (human β defensins—HBD 1 and 2, cathelicidins and granulysin) which also contribute to inflammation and follicular rupture.
5. *P. acnes* is known to produce biofilms (a complex aggregation of microorganisms with an extracellular polysaccharide lining) which promote bacterial resistance to antimicrobial agents. Virulence factors are produced which help sustain the organism in a hostile environment.

GENETIC FACTORS IN ACNE

Genetic factors have been incriminated to be an important etiologic factor. Twin studies (monozygotic and dizygotic) and familial studies have shown the incidence to be rather high in identical twins and that acne can run in families.

Several genes have been studied to identify the role of genetic factors (Fig. 1.4).

a. *Genes of steroid metabolism:* Human cytochrome P-450A1 (CYP1A1), steroid 17α-hydroxylase, 17, 20-lyase activity, steroid 21-hydroxylase gene (CYP21) and androgen receptor (AR) genes are some of the genes under scrutiny.
b. *Genes for IGF-1:* Since elevated levels of IGF-1 correlate with overproduction of sebum and acne, genetic polymorphisms in the IGF-1 gene are being studied.
c. *Innate immunity genes:* Mutation in the TLR2 and TLR4 genes, IL-1α gene are of current interest in research circles.
d. *Genes of autoimmune inflammatory syndromes:* Acne is a component of autoinflammatory syndromes like PAPA (pyogenic arthritis, pyoderma gangrenosum and acne) and SAPHO (synovitis, acne, pustulosis, hyperostosis, osteitis) syndromes.

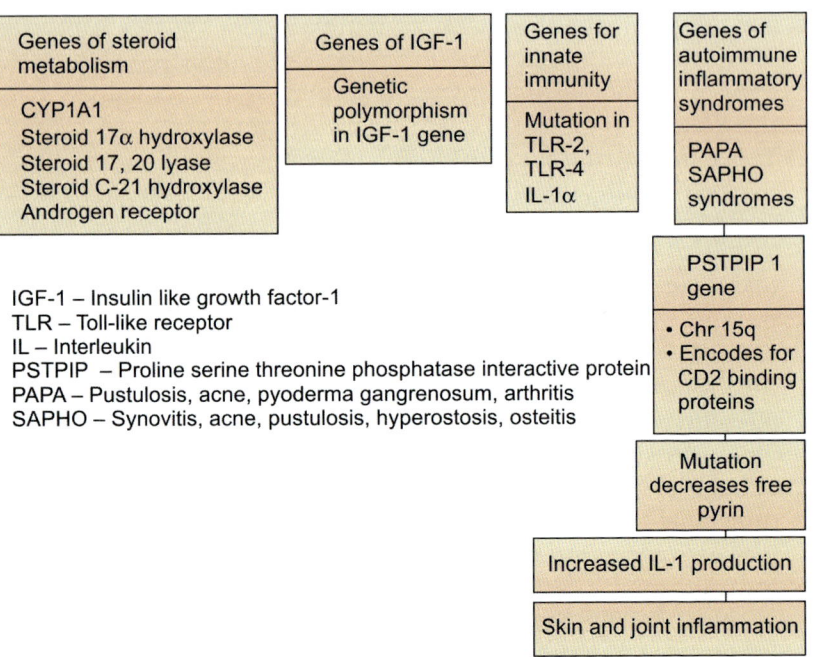

Genes of steroid metabolism	Genes of IGF-1	Genes for innate immunity	Genes of autoimmune inflammatory syndromes
CYP1A1 Steroid 17α hydroxylase Steroid 17, 20 lyase Steroid C-21 hydroxylase Androgen receptor	Genetic polymorphism in IGF-1 gene	Mutation in TLR-2, TLR-4 IL-1α	PAPA SAPHO syndromes

IGF-1 – Insulin like growth factor-1
TLR – Toll-like receptor
IL – Interleukin
PSTPIP – Proline serine threonine phosphatase interactive protein
PAPA – Pustulosis, acne, pyoderma gangrenosum, arthritis
SAPHO – Synovitis, acne, pustulosis, hyperostosis, osteitis

PSTPIP 1 gene
• Chr 15q
• Encodes for CD2 binding proteins

Mutation decreases free pyrin

Increased IL-1 production

Skin and joint inflammation

Fig. 1.4: Genetic factors in acne: Several genetic components are being studied to identify genetic propensity to acne

The PSTPIP1 gene (proline-serine-threonine-phosphatase interactive protein 1) is encoded on chromosome 15q and encodes for CD2 binding protein (CD2BP1). Pyrin, an inhibitor of inflammation, is normally bound to PSTPIP1. In mutations of this gene there is an increased binding of PSTPIP to pyrin. This results in decreased free pyrin available, which in turn, increases caspase-1 recruitment and thus increased IL-1 production. IL-1 produces inflammation of the skin and joints.

ENVIRONMENTAL FACTORS

The role of environmental factors as a trigger for acne has generated interest lately. The primary factors identified include diet, stress, smoking, seasonal influences and use of cosmetics and occlusive toiletries (Fig. 1.5).

1. Diet

A general consensus on the role of diet in acne pathogenesis has never been achieved as scientific studies have been conflicting in their outcomes. Until recently it was felt that diet does not influence acne at all, and that anecdotal reports are to be shunned. There were also

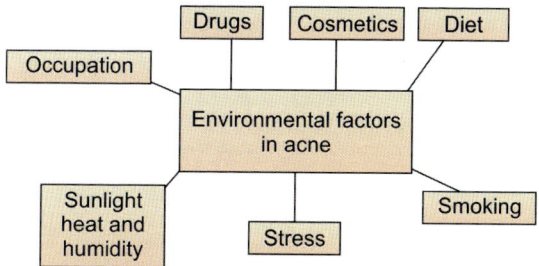

Fig. 1.5: Various extraneous factors that can influence acne vulgaris

doubts raised about the design of the studies that identified a positive correlation between acne and dietary influences.

Recently, much interest has been generated in this regard, based on the role identified for IGF-1 and the growth hormone, in acne pathogenesis. These elements are considered as important as androgens, if not greater.

The role for IGF-1 and growth hormone is substantiated by the following observations:

• A spurt in acne correlates with the spurt in the levels of growth hormone in puberty. Growth hormone binds to its receptor in the peripheral body cells and induces IGF-1 in the liver. IGF-1 is a key regulator of growth. IGF-1 stimulates 5-alpha reductase enzyme, induces adrenal and gonadal androgen synthesis, androgen receptor signal transduction and sebocyte proliferation and lipogenesis.
• IGF-1 is strongly expressed in the mature sebocytes and suprabasal cells of the sebaceous ducts.
• Congenital IGF-1 deficient individuals (Laron syndrome) have no acne.
• High glycemic foods implicated in acne are known to have increase IGF-1 levels and serum insulin levels.
• Patients with insulin resistance, obesity, polycystic ovaries, acro-megaly, and skimmed milk consumption are known to express high levels of IGF-1 and increased sebaceous gland activity.

Foods with low glycemic index (GI) tend to lower the levels of acne while high glycemic foods, which are characteristic of the western diet, tends to increase acne levels. Ethnic groups living in non westernised Papua New Guinea and Paraguay rely on a low glycemic food like fruits, lean protein and healthy fats have a little or no acne.

On the contrary, a western diet is seen to have an influence on the incidence of acne, especially in those that have migrated to western civilizations. Milk, though a low glycemic diet, is known to aggravate acne, especially if consumed as skimmed milk. This is attributed to

Protective diets	Aggravational diets
Mediterranean diet	High glycemic load
Fish	Dairy food
Omega 3 fatty acid rich diets	High fat diet
Fruits	Chocolates
Foods rich in antioxidants and zinc	Nuts
Dietary fibre	Skimmed milk
	Ice creams
	Iodine rich diet (seaweed consumption in *Korea*)

the whey protein content and the casein content in milk, which have been identified to have an insulinotropic effect. Casein is known to stimulate IGF-1 more than whey protein.

The mechanism by which glycemic loads modulate acne is not well known. It is postulated that low GI foods influence sebum composition by decreasing glycogen stores in sebaceous glands which would limit sebum lipogenesis and decrease insulin levels. This would in turn reduce testosterone bioavailability and DHEA-S concentrations.

Based on current data there is convincing evidence of high glycemic foods and dairy products exacerbating acne. Further elucidation of the roles of diet on androgen metabolism and sensitivity as well as on IGF-1 would make the picture clearer.

2. Cigarette Smoking

The effects of smoking on acne have been controversial as in the case of dietary influences. Six studies have favoured a negative or no association, whereas four studies have shown a positive association.

It has been postulated that nicotine present in cigarettes can bind to acetylcholine receptors (AChR) present on the sebaceous gland and exert an anti-inflammatory effect. This has given rise to the hypothesis that "smokers acne" has a lesser incidence of inflammatory and greater incidence of comedonal acne as ACh is thought to increase follicular hyperkeratinisation at high concentrations.

3. Sunlight, Heat and Humidity

The role of sunlight in aggravating acne has been controversial too. Patients report exacerbation in summer months and with heat and humidity (personal observation) and an entity called acne aestivalis has been reported with hot temperatures. However, patients also report improvement of acne on exposure to sunlight. A positive influence has also been noted with PUVA, NB-UVB, red, blue and full spectrum light, thus making light a useful adjunct to therapy of acne. This dichotomy is yet to be understood.

STRESS

Stress is a well-known trigger for acne. A classic example has been examination associated stress leading onto acute "break outs" in students. The study by Chiu et al on 22 universities students has shown a direct association between stress and acne after having controlled

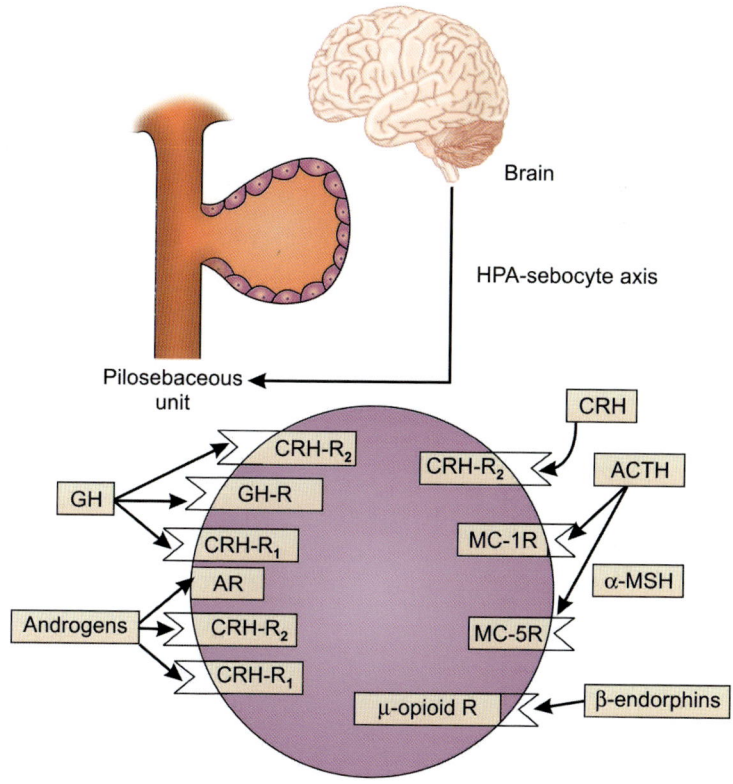

HPA axis – Hypothalamopituitary adrenal axis
CRH – Corticotropin-releasing hormone
ACTH – Adrenocorticotropin hormone
MSH – Melanocyte-stimulating hormone
GH – Growth hormone
MC and MC-R – Melanocortin, melanocortin-receptor

Fig. 1.6: The sebocyte is a hotbed of neuro-immuno-endocrine activity. Receptors are present in the sebocyte for CRH, ACTH, α-MSH and β-endorphins. They are collectively called melanocortins and mediate their action through melanocortin (MC) receptors (MC-R). This explains the role stress plays in exacerbation of acne

for changes in diet habits and sleep. Patient reported observations on exacerbation with stress related events in life add credence to the influence of the emotional segment of the brain on the skin.

The exact mechanism is not well understood. Increased levels of glucocorticoids and adrenal androgens that are released during periods of emotional stress are the dominant pathogenetic factors identified (Fig. 1.6). Receptors are present on the sebaceous glands for CRH, MSH and steroids. These hormones are known to be closely associated with emotionally stressed situations.

CONCLUSION

The pathogenesis of acne is multifactorial. Traditional concepts of this being a purely androgen mediated disease have changed. Acne is a complex disease influenced by an altered sebaceous gland milieu that leads to a train of immunopathologic events culminating in comedogenesis, inflammation and tissue scarring.

SUGGESTED READINGS

1. Acneiform eruptions in dermatology. A differential diagnosis. Joshua A Zeichner(Ed). Springer
2. Deplewski D and Rosenfield RL. Role of hormones in pilosebaceous unit development. Endocr Rev. 2000; 21(4):363–92. Review.
3. Thiboutot D. Acne: Hormonal concepts and therapy. Clin Dermatol. 2004; 22(5):419–28.
4. Thiboutot D. Hormones and acne: Pathophysiology, clinical evaluation and therapies. Semin Cutan Med Surg. 2001; 20(3):144–53.
5. White GM. Recent findings in the epidemiologic evidence, classification and subtypes of acne vulgaris. J Am Acad Dermatol. 1998; 39:S34–7.
6. World Clinics Dermatology: Acne. Dec 2013, Vol1: 1. Neena Khanna (Ed).

2

Identifying the Acne Patient

INTRODUCTION

Acne starts in adolescence and frequently resolves by the mid-twenties. A peak in prevalence and severity occurs between 14 and 17 years in females, when 40% are affected, and 16 to 19 years in males, when 35% are affected [Burton JL, 1971]. A study from the USA indicated that the prevalence by the mid-teens was virtually 100%.

In patients with very mild disease the problem is referred to as physiological acne. Acne develops earlier in females than in males which may be indicative of earlier onset of puberty. Significant prepubertal acne is only rarely found to be a cutaneous marker of an endocrine abnormality but should be considered in early-onset acne. Site of involvement is linked to the age of onset of the disease, with inflammatory lesions in the midline of the face presenting early in sexual maturation.

The resolution of acne is a matter of debate and though by 20 to 25 years the tendency is for acne to resolve [Cunliffe WJ, 1979], in 7–17% of individuals clinical acne persists beyond the age of 25 years [Goulden V, 1997], with physiological acne in females having a prevalence of 24%. Countries with widespread use of OCPs, have noted a decrease in the prevalence of acne in females [Jemec GBE, 2002]. But there are authors that have reported the persistence of acne. Most have acne persisting from adolescence, but 8% have late-onset (age over 25 years) acne. At the age of 40 years, significant lesions are still present in 1% of males and 5% of females. Is this because of a more referrals to dermatologists or an indication of hormonal acne; is a question of debate. Factors that underlie the resolution of acne are not understood, nor are their relative persistence in females. Recent studies on the natural history of acne are limited, because improved treatment has modified the prevalence, severity and age of presentation to dermatological clinics.

CLINICAL MORPHOLOGY

Acne is classically described as a polymorphic disorder and most patients have a mixture of lesions. Non-inflammed lesions are the earliest lesions to develop in younger patients and include both open (blackheads) and closed (whiteheads) comedones.

Open comedones represent dome-shaped papules in which there are dilated follicular outlets filled with keratin. The apparent black colour is thought to be due to melanin deposited within the cellular debris (Fig. 2.1).

Closed comedones or whiteheads are generally 1 mm in diameter, skin coloured and have no visible follicular opening. These lesions are often inconspicuous and require adequate lighting and stretching of the skin to be seen (Fig. 2.2).

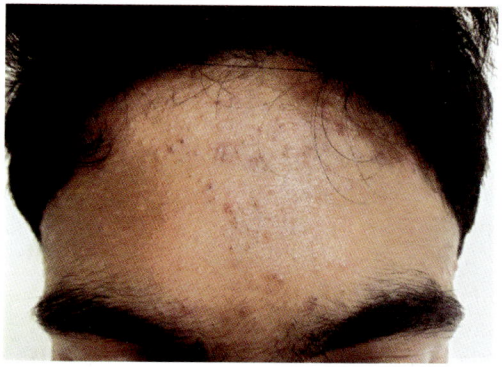

Fig. 2.1: A male patient with predominant "black heads" or open comedone on the forehead. Such lesions are largely non-inflammatory and are easily treated by topical retinoids

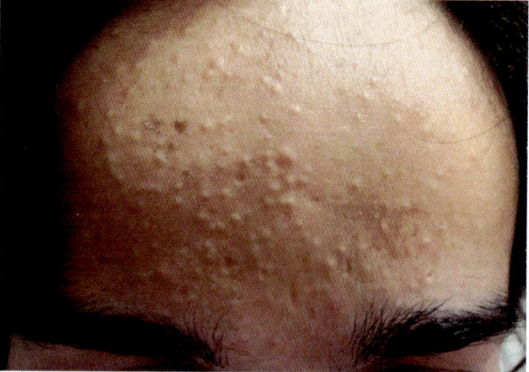

Fig. 2.2: Multiple white heads or closed comedones, resembling "sand paper". These are difficult to treat and some dermatologists use low energy RF or Up CO_2 to treat these lesions

Missed comedones will be visualized on stretching the skin, and using a good light, at a shallow angle, in about 20% of patients, which would have been otherwise missed and therefore not treated.

'Sandpaper' comedones consist of multiple, very small white-heads, frequently distributed on the forehead (Fig. 2.2), which produce a roughened, gritty feel to the skin.

'Macrocomedones' are large whiteheads or occasionally blackheads greater than 1 mm in diameter. Both macrocomedones and sandpaper comedones respond poorly to conventional topical treatments.

'Submarine' comedones are large comedonal structures greater than 0.5 cm in diameter and are deeply entrenched and lead to inflammatory nodular lesions (Fig. 2.3).

Secondary comedones are consequent to exposure to dioxins (chloracne), pomades (pomade acne), topical steroids and other drugs (drug-induced acne).

Inflammatory lesions arise from the microcomedone or non-inflammatory lesions and can develop into superficial or deep lesions. The superficial lesions are usually papules and pustules (5 mm or less in diameter) and the deep lesions are deep pustules and nodules. A major textbook states that the term nodulo-cystic acne is incorrect as acne 'cysts' are not true cysts because they are not lined by an epithelium. It is therefore more accurate to describe such lesions as nodules.

Scarring usually follows deep-seated inflammatory lesions, but may also occur as a result of more superficial inflamed lesions in scar-prone patients. Close inspection under a bright light may reveal some scarring, albeit mild, in up to 90% of patients who attend a dermato-logist. Scars may show increased collagen (hypertrophic scars and

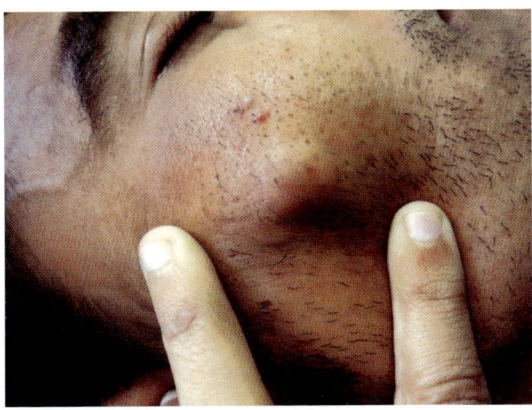

Fig. 2.3: Submarine comedones are deep lesions and are difficult to treat and diagnose

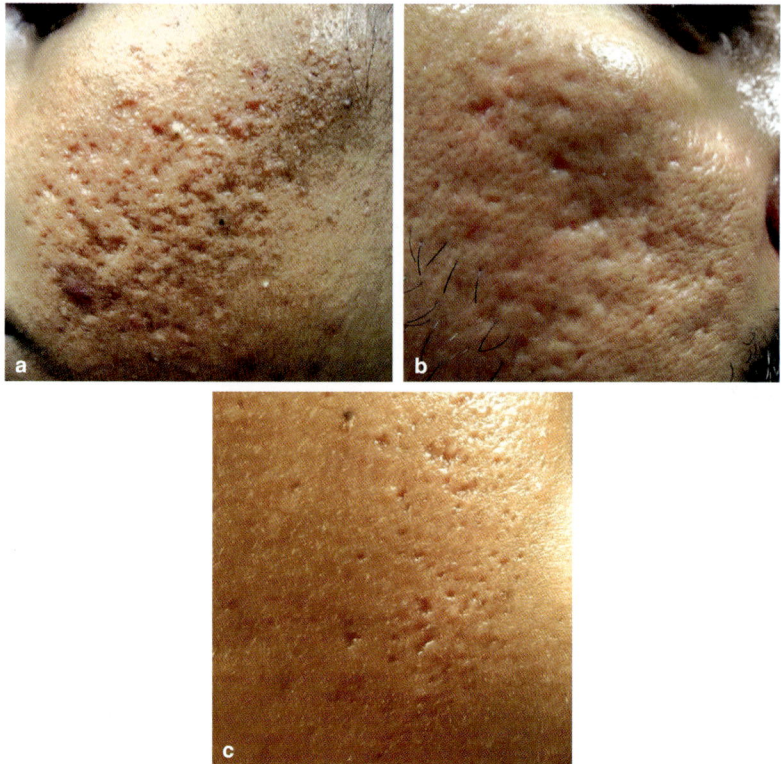

Fig. 2.4: Different types of acne scars (a) large scars with vertical edges "box car", (b) rolling scars and (c) deep V-shaped scars "ice-pick scars"

keloids) or be associated with loss of collagen (i.e. ice-pick scars, depressed fibrotic scars, atrophic macules and perifollicular elastolysis). A depiction of common scars is elegantly demonstrated in Fig. 2.4a to c.

Another way to describe clinical features is to classify them into grades as mild, moderate and severe.

MILD ACNE VULGARIS

These are predominantly composed of *comedones, papules and pustules.*

Biopsy sections of normal-looking skin in patients with comedonal acne may show histological features of microcomedones in 28% of cases (Cunliffe WJ, 2004). The fact that the microcomedone is the initial acne lesion highlights the need of applying topical acne therapies not only on clinically apparent lesions but also on the *whole* face.

Of the comedones described above a few are important to identify as their therapy can be challenging.

Sandpaper comedones: These lesions are a therapeutic challenge as they are difficult to treat, may become inflamed, and show a little or variable response to oral antibiotics and topical retinoids. Best results are obtained with treatment with oral isotretinoin at a dose of 0.5 mg/kg/day (Cunliffe WJ, 2001).

Macrocomedones: These do not respond to conventional therapy and light electrofulguration is needed in most cases.

MILD AND MODERATE INFLAMMATORY ACNE VULGARIS

This phenotype is probably the most common type presenting to the clinician.

Inflammatory acne lesions may be macules, papules, pustules, or nodules. Acne can be primarily papular, pustular, or nodular according to the predominant lesions, but there may be an equal number of comedones and papules (comedopapular acne) or papules and pustules (papulopustular acne).

Acne papulopustulosa should be differentiated from other acneiform dermatoses, including drug-induced acne, gram-negative folliculitis, acne aestivalis (mallorca acne), and papulopustular rosacea (Fig. 2.5).

Acneiform dermatoses are follicular reactions and not variants of acne vulgaris. They present clinically with monomorphous inflammatory lesions, usually papules or pustules. Comedones are uncommon. *Drug-induced* acne may be caused by corticosteroids, anabolic steroids, corticotropin, vitamins B1, B6, B12, D2, anticonvulsants, lithium, isoniazid, quinidine, cyclosporine, iodides, and bromides [Plewig G, 1998]. The patient's history of drug intake, the sudden onset and the

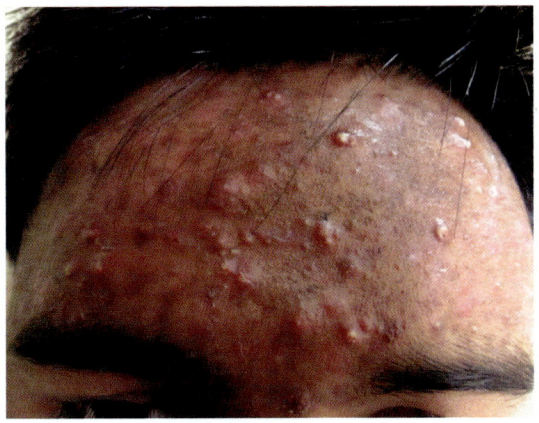

Fig. 2.5: An admixture of papules, pustules, nodules and pigmentation (moderate grade acne)

monomorphous nature of the lesions, the absence of comedones, and the localization on the trunk and the upper extremities should lead to correct diagnosis.

Gram-negative folliculitis is caused by overgrowth of gram-negative species due to long-term oral antibiotic intake and may be considered in the case of treatment failure or acne flare-up during antibiotic therapy.

Acne aestivalis presents after sun exposure and consists of multiple papular lesions, on the sides of the neck, the chest, shoulders, upper arms, and occasionally cheeks.

SEVERE ACNE VULGARIS

This is the type where aggressive therapy is needed as in most cases scarring ensues.

The first subtype is characterized by presence of numerous nodules and cysts, while more than 40 comedones, papules, and pustules are also present (Fig. 2.6).

Acne conglobata is an uncommon form of acne vulgaris that presents with numerous comedones, papules, pustules, nodules, abscesses, and draining sinus tracts involving mainly the chest, back, and buttocks. Patients with acne conglobata are predominantly males with extensive acne characterized by severe nodular inflammation and scarring. A *hallmark* of this disease is the presence of grouped comedones, mainly on the posterior neck and upper trunk . Draining sinuses may be seen in the form of a persistent lesion of linear or angular shape with a discharge of pus or blood. It persists for years, with no tendency to spontaneous resolution. Acne conglobata may occur in association with hidradenitis suppurativa as part of the follicular occlusion triad (acne

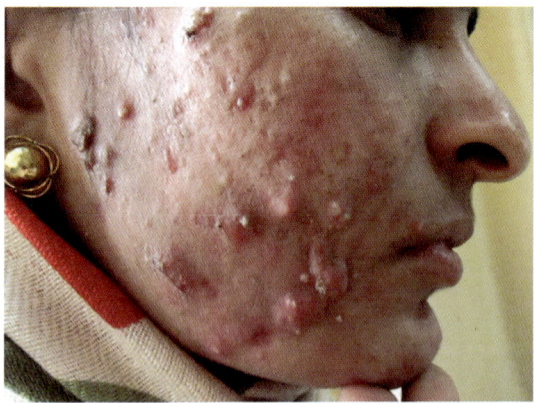

Fig. 2.6: A female patient with nodules and cysts. Such case should warrant an investigation for an underlying hormonal disorder

conglobata, hidradenitis sup-purativa, and dissecting cellulitis of the scalp).

ADULT ACNE

It has been a conventional and dogmatic teaching that acne vulgaris is a disorder that usually appears at puberty and resolves in late adolescence or early adult life. In fact, there are a significant number of adults who also suffer from acne. Adult acne can be divided into *persistent* acne which continues into adult life from the teen years and *adult-onset acne* which first appears after age of 25 years. The prevalence of adult acne ranges in women from 12 to 51% and in men from 3 to 42%. It is safe to conclude that adults with acne are not rare and that women tend to have a higher prevalence than men. Of all the factors that may predispose to such a trend possibly a hormonal influence seems to be marked.

Hormonal Influences on Adult Acne

It is possible that the mechanisms involved in the pathogenesis of adolescent, persistent, and late-onset acne may be different [Till AE, 2000]. Special mention should be made of the role of hormones in adults with acne. There are studies that have shown that men with mild forms of congenital adrenal hyper-plasia (CAH) and elevated androgens are acne prone [Placzek M, 2005]. But the link between hormones and acne is usually significant in adult women with acne.

There are numerous series documenting elevated free testosterone (T), dihydrotestosterone (DHT), and/or dehydroepiandrosterone sulfate (DHEAS), as well as low sex hormone binding globulin (SHBG) in both persistent and late-onset adult acne. In many studies, the individual serum levels of androgens have been found to be abnormal; in other studies, individual serum levels of hormones are normal, but mean androgen levels are higher in the patients with acne [Aizawa H, 1993 and Darley CR, 1984].

The clinical finding of a clinical flare of acne in the premenstrual phase of the menstrual cycle is a proof of concept of the hormonal link in acne. A study of women 18–44 years of age with acne showed that 63% had documented premenstrual inflammatory acne flares [Lucky AW, 2004]. Although possibly caused by elevated androgens, another hypothesis for the etiology of the premenstrual flare is a relatively lower mid-cycle peak of estrogen in women with acne.

Correlation of adult acne to signs and symptoms of polycystic ovary syndrome (PCOS), as well as other hyperandrogenic disorders such as congenital adrenal hyperplasia (CAH) and Cushing disease, is also well documented and supports the role of hormone abnormalities in adults with these conditions. Postmenopausal acne has been postulated to occur because of the influence of residual adrenal and ovarian androgens acting unopposed by estrogen.

An end-organ cutaneous abnormality of androgen metabolism, in particular the conversion of T to DHT by type 5-α-reductase in acne-prone follicles, is also likely to be important [Thiboutot D, 2003]. Genetic factors may determine abnormal follicular keratinization or sebaceous gland androgen response in individuals with persistent acne and now an increasing role of insulin-like growth factor-1 (IGF-1) levels, the levels of which may influence sebum production and acne in adult men and women [Cappel M, 2005].

Clinical Manifestations

Adult acne may be either persistent or late onset: Persistent acne represents a continuum from adolescence into adult life, whereas late-onset acne has been defined as occurring for the first time after the age of 25 years.

While early *pubertal* acne initially occurs on the forehead and proceeds down the central part of the face [Lucky AW, 1994], *adult* women tend to have acne on the lower third of the face, especially on the chin and in the perioral region (Figs 2.7 and 2.8) [Vexiau P, 1990]. In adult women, deep-seated inflammatory papules and nodules are most common [Poli F, 2001]. A premenstrual flare of deep papules or nodules in the late luteal phase of the menstrual cycle is a common complaint in many adult women. In some women, acne may persist throughout the menstrual cycle. Acne can also occur sporadically and affect the trunk, especially in postmenopausal women.

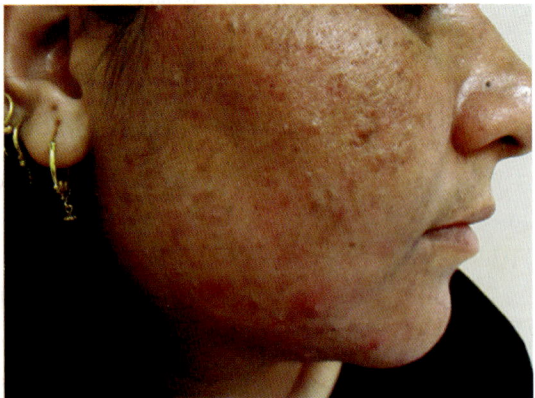

Fig. 2.7: Case of persistent acne, note the involvement of the jaw line

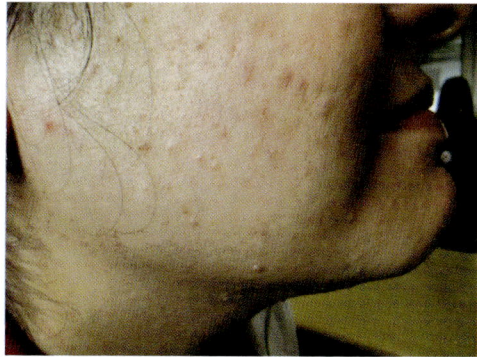

Fig. 2.8: A persistent acne case with lesions on the face and jaw line

Treatment

Though this will be detailed subsequently, hormonal therapy and isotretinoin are the mainstays of treatment.

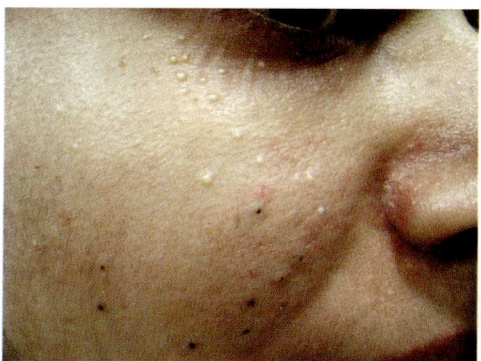

Fig. 2.9: A case of acne with milia on the face

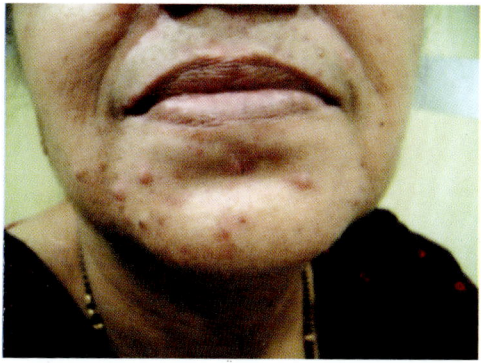

Fig. 2.10: Perioral dermatitis in a female patients

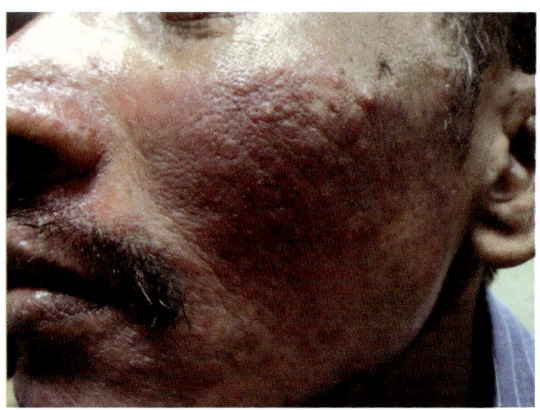

Fig. 2.11: A case of seborrhoeic dermatitis with rosacea

There are some common conditions that mimic acne and some of these are depicted in Figs 2.9 to 2.11.

REFERENCES

1. Aizawa H, Miimura M. Adrenal androgen abnormalities in women with late onset and persistent acne. Arch Dermatol Res. 1993; 284:451–5.

2. Burton JL, Cunliffe WJ, Stafford L et al. The prevalence of acne vulgaris in adolescence. Br J Dermatol 1971; 85:119–26.

3. Cappel M, Mauger D, Thiboutot D. Correlation between serum levels of insulin-like growth factor-1, dehydroepiandrosterone sulfate, and dihydrotestosterone and acne lesions counts in adult women. Arch Dermatol. 2005; 141:333–8.

4. Cunliffe WJ, Gollnick H. Acne diagnosis and management. London: Martin Dunitz, Ltd; 2001. Clin Dermatol. 2004;22:367–74.

5. Cunliffe WJ, Gould DJ. Prevalence of facial acne vulgaris in late adolescence and in adults. BMJ 1979; 1:1109–10.

6. Cunliffe WJ, Holland DB, Jeremy A. Comedone formation: Etiology, clinical presentation, and treatment Clin Dermatol. 2004 Sep-Oct;22(5):367–74. Review.

7. Darley CR, Moore JW, Besser GM, et al. Androgen status in women with late onset or persistent acne vulgaris. Clin Exp Dermatol. 1984; 9:28–35.

8. Goulden V, Clark SM, Cunliffe WJ. Postadolescent acne: A review of clinical features. Br J Dermatol 1997; 136:66–70.

9. Jemec GBE, Linneberg A, Nielsen NH et al. Have oral contraceptives reduced the prevalence of acne? A population-based study of acne vulgaris, tobacco smoking and oral contraceptives. Dermatology 2002; 204:179–84.

10. Lucky AW. Quantitative Documentation of a Premenstrual Flare of Facial Acne in Adult Women. Arch Dermatol. 2004; 140:423–4.

11. Lucky AW, Biro FM, Huster GA, et al. Acne vulgaris in premenarchal girls. Arch Dermatol. 1994; 130(3):308–14.

12. Placzek M, Arnold B, Schmidt H, et al. Elevated 17-hydroxyproge-sterone serum values in male patients with acne. J Am Acad Dermatol. 2005; 53:955–8.

13. Plewig G, Jansen T. Acneiform dermatoses. Dermatology. 1998; 196:102–7.

14. Poli F, Dreno B, Verschoore M. An epidemiological study of acne in female adults: Results of a survey conducted in France. JEADV. 2001; 15:541–5.

15. Thiboutot D, Chen W. Update and future of hormonal therapy in acne. Dermatology. 2003; 206:57–67.

16. Till AE, Goulden V, Cunliffe WJ, et al. The cutaneous microflora of adolescent, persistent and late-onset patients does not differ. Br J Dermatol. 2000; 142:885–92.

17. Vexiau P, Husson C, Chivot M, et al. Androgen excess in women with acne alone compared with women with acne and/or hirsutism. J Invest Dermatol. 1990; 94:279–83.

3

How and When to Investigate

INTRODUCTION

The investigations that are required in acne vulgaris are many and can be used for diagnosis and treatment. As most clinicians wrongly consider acne as a "rite of passage" which all have to bear, it is rarely investigated.

In cases of persistent acne in females and sometimes in males endogenous hormonal causes may play a role. This chapter will focus on this aspect and PCOS which is a common cause of hormonal acne.

Polycystic Ovary Syndrome

PCOS, is the most common endocrinopathy in women of reproductive age, is characterized by oligo/amenorrhea, clinical features of hyper-androgenism (i.e. acne, alopecia, hirsutism) and/or biochemical hyperandrogenemia, and/or polycystic ovaries. Biochemical hyper-androgenemia is most frequently detected with measurement of *free testosterone*, which is elevated in ~70% of cases. Expert groups recommend that secondary causes of the presenting symptoms be excluded before PCOS is diagnosed. These include non-classic CAH, hyperprolactinemia, and androgen-secreting tumors.

Adrenal Causes

Congenital Adrenal Hyperplasia

CAH, a group of autosomal recessive disorders of steroid biosynthesis, is most commonly caused by deficiencies in 21-hydroxylase (90% to 95% of cases) and 11-hydroxylase (5 to 8% of cases). Rare enzyme deficiencies are also seen in 3β-hydroxysteroid dehydrogenase and 17-hydroxylase. Overlapping clinical features make the differential diagnosis of CAH difficult. However, measuring steroid profiles rather than single steroids has improved the diagnostic accuracy.

Late-onset CAH is commonly caused by 21-hydroxylase deficiency and rarely by 11-hydroxylase deficiency. Both present in childhood or post-puberty with evidence of androgen excess (e.g. hirsutism, oligomenorrhea).

Screening for late-onset 21-hydroxylase deficiency requires an early morning (before 8 am) serum collection for 17-hydroxyprogesterone. Levels > 170–200 ng/dL suggest 21-hydroxylase deficiency and require follow-up testing after cosyntropin stimulation with either a complete adrenocortical steroid profile in children or a 17-hydroxyprogesterone test in adults. An increased baseline 11-deoxycortisol and/or deoxycorticosterone level suggests 11-hydroxylase deficiency. An exaggerated increase in either of these steroids after cosyntropin stimulation can confirm the diagnosis.

Premature Adrenarche

Premature adrenarche refers to an abnormal increase in adrenal androgen production that results in the appearance of pubic and/or axillary hair before age 8 in girls and age 9 in boys. This condition is much more common in girls than boys (10:1). In girls, premature adrenarche is not benign and is associated with increased incidence of PCOS, metabolic syndrome, and type II diabetes mellitus later in life. The impact of premature adrenarche in boys is inconclusive. In premature adrenarche, androgens such as androstenedione, dehydroepiandrosterone (DHEA), and testosterone are moderately increased for chronological age.

Markedly increased testosterone levels (> 150 ng/dL) are associated with androgen-secreting tumours.

HISTORY

Persistent and late-onset acne is distinguished by whether acne was continuous since adolescence or first appeared after age 25 years. Family history often reveals a familial predilection to acne with first-degree relatives affected. Many women will complain of menstrual irregularities, usually oligomenorrhea. The salient clinical features that necessitate investigations for an underlying hormonal cause are given in Table 3.1.

Table 3.1 *Clinical presentations that dictate investigations*		
Clinical features	*Clinical scenario*	*Signs of hyperandrogenism*
Multiple comedones	Severe/sudden acne	Irregular menses
Hyperseborrhoea	Therapy-resistant acne	Hirsutism
Mature onset/perioral distribution	Rapid significant relapse post-isotretinoin	Hyperseborrhoea

It is my experience that a proportion of patients, specially females have cosmetic induced acne, thus an inquiry of topical preparations such as moisturizers, sunscreens, foundations and facials are important. Inquiry about oral medications, especially those started within a few months of the onset of acne, is needed. Patients should be asked about use of progestin—only contraceptives or androgenic OCP, before thinking about underlying hormonal causes for acne.

PHYSICAL EXAMINATION

Concomitant findings of hirsutism and female pattern hair loss strongly suggest hyperandrogenemia. True virilization with clitoromegaly, deepening voice, or increased muscle mass is rarer and suggestive of an androgen secreting tumour. Acanthosis nigricans and obesity with an increased waist-hip ratio are often signs of the metabolic syndrome.

Acne involving the "U" area of the face, jawline, recalcitrant to therapy including isotretinoin and premenstrual flare is suggestive of hormonal acne.

LABORATORY EVALUATION

In *most* cases of acne, an investigation is not required. Unless patients with acne show other features of hyperandrogenism, it is not necessary to investigate for an endocrinopathy. But in cases recalcitrant to therapy, it is important to rule out other causes.

An endocrine evaluation requires a lab investigation early in the menstrual cycle (day 1–3). If late-onset congenital adrenal hyperplasia is suspected, then a 09.00 am cortisol and 17α-hydroxyprogesterone measurement should be performed. It is *very rare* to find virilizing tumours that present as acne alone. When thought necessary, appropriate initial tests should include measurement of total testosterone, SHBG, androstenedione, AMH, FAI, dehydroepiandrosterone (DHEA), prolactin, follicle-stimulating hormone (FSH) and luteinizing hormone (LH).

In women, elevated serum testosterone levels can be due to androgen-secreting tumours of the adrenal gland or ovary (>150 ng/dL), PCOS, late-onset congenital adrenal hyperplasia, or Cushing syndrome. Testosterone results should be interpreted in conjunction with other laboratory and clinical findings. Medical conditions altering serum concentrations of SHBG or albumin may affect the bioavailable testosterone level. Albumin levels *decrease* with liver disease, kidney disease, and nutritional deficiency, whereas SHBG levels *decrease* with obesity, diabetes mellitus, chronic illness, hypothyroidism, and use of glucocorticoids, progestins, and androgenic steroids. SHBG levels *increase* with aging in men, liver disease, hyperthyroidism, and use of anticonvulsants and estrogens.

A overview of the investigations and their interpretation is given in Table 3.2.

Table 3.2 *Investigations required to identify an endocrine problem in acne*		
Androgen profile	Testosterone (>150–200 ng /dl) and SHBG Androgen index (>2.5/5) 17(OH)-progesterone (>170 ng/dl) DHEAS (>400 µg/dl) FSH, LH (>2) AMH (>6.8 ng/ml)/(3.34 ng/ml)	PCOS: Mild increase Tumour >200 ng/dl Hyperandrogenism NCCAH >400 µg/dl: PCOS, CAH >800 µg/dl: Tumours, Cushing's syndrome PCOS
Imaging studies	**USG** (>12 follicles between 2 and 9 mm in diameter or ovarian volume > 10 cm³) USG is sensitive but not specific (occurs in CAH and Cushing's syndrome). Usually transvaginal but transabdominal possible in experienced hands **CT scan**	PCOS, Tumours
Adrenal gland	**S. cortisol, Dexamethasone suppression test**	It helps to identify congenital adrenal hyperplasia along with DHEAS and 17(OH) progesterone
Metabolic	**Insulin Level (> 10 IU) /HOMO-IR index (>2.5)** **S. lipid profile**	Insulin resistance Metabolic syndrome
Others	Prolactin/thyroid function tests Urinary free cortisol or overnight dexamethasone suppression test IGF-1	Mild increase in prolactin in PCOS Cushing's syndrome Acromegaly

PCOS

Polycystic ovarian syndrome is the most frequently associated hormonal disease [Bunker CB, 1989]. In most acne clinics, the majority of female patients with acne have no other clinical features of the syndrome, which consists of hirsutism, relative infertility or irregular menstruation. Though, there is no correlation between the presence of ovarian cysts and the severity of the acne [Peserico A, 1989].

An ovarian source of excess androgen can be suspected in cases where the serum total testosterone is elevated (>100 ng/dl). A raised serum testosterone and an increased LH level are seen in patients with polycystic ovarian disease. The LH : FSH ratio is *not* always elevated in PCOS and is not necessarily a diagnostic measure. But a value >2 is considered to be suggestive of PCOS.

Another option is to use AMH as a tool to diagnose both hyper-androgenism and PCOS. Since AMH is produced directly by the ovarian follicles, AMH levels correlate with the number of antral follicles in the ovaries. It has been documented that women to lower AMH have lower antral follicular counts and produce a lower number of oocytes compared with women with higher levels. AMH levels do not change significantly throughout the menstrual cycle and decrease with age. Healthy women, below 38 years old, with normal follicular status at day 3 of the menstrual cycle, have AMH levels of 2.0–6.8 ng/ml (14.28–48.55 pmol/l). High levels are found in patients with PCOS (> 6.8 ng/ml). Different labs have different cut off and 3.4 ng/ml is another cut off that has been found in a study from India.

We use the AMH level as it is a much better marker for ovarian reserve. It is much more stable than the FSH level and does not vary from cycle to cycle. Even better, it can be measured on any day of the cycle. One confusing thing about AMH is that there are at least 2 scales out there and innumerable clinic definitions of what is "normal"—it depends on which assay they use and which study! One scale is ng/ml and one is pmol/l. The pmol/l scale runs from 0 to about 48; the ng/ml runs from 0 to about 10. On the ng/ml scale, less than 2 ng/ml is considered to be low. A value of 2.2–4.0 ng/ml is satisfactory, 4.0–6.8 is optimal and more than that indicates PCOS. The Rotterdam criteria for PCOS (antral follicle count (AFC) ≥12 and/or ovarian volume >10 ml) has been revised by increasing the AFC >20 and an AMH-based threshold of >35 pmol/l. A large number of studies have found it to be a useful tool for diagnosing PCOS and hyperandrogenism [Parahuleva N, 2014; Pinola P, 2014; Wiweko B, 2014; Lauritsen MP, 2014], though, age-sex matched, studies are needed to validate it in Indian populations. In my practice, I find it to be a useful tool to diagnose a case of PCOS.

ADRENAL ANDROGENS/CAH

Late-onset adrenal hyperplasia due to a partial deficiency of 21-hydroxylase should be considered in patients with persistent problems with their acne [McLaughlin B, 1990] and may rarely cause severe acne in boys [Placzek M, 1999]. Either the adrenal gland or the ovary may produce excess androgens. Serum dehydroepiandrosterone sulphate (DHEAS) levels can be used to screen for an adrenal source of excess androgen production, patients with a serum DHEAS greater than 800 µg/dL may have an adrenal tumour. Some adrenal tumours may also produce testosterone. Values of DHEAS in the range of 370–803 µg/dL may be seen with congenital adrenal hyperplasia, which is often associated with a slightly raised cortisol and a 17α-hydroxyprogesterone level of greater than 170 ng/dl. To confirm congenital adrenal hyperplasia non-classical form (NCCAH), the ACTH stimulation test is required.

The gold standard for diagnosis of NCCAH remains the ACTH (cosyntropin) stimulation test. Baseline samples are collected for 17-OHP and cortisol after which synthetic ACTH (cosyntropin) is administered with a standard dose of 250 µg for older children and adults. Repeat blood work is collected 60 minutes after administration to determine the stimulated values of both 17-OHP and cortisol. While stimulated 17-OHP levels with classic CAH typically exceed 20,000 ng/dl, those with NCCAH will have 17-OHP levels within the range of 1,500–10,000 ng/dl poststimulation. Cortisol levels are collected to document adrenal reserve.

In clinical practice, it is *not* feasible to administer ACTH stimulation tests on all individuals suspected of having NCCAH who in fact have clinical symptomatology that closely mirror that of PCOS or other androgenic conditions. Instead, it has been proposed to use baseline non-stimulated values of 17-OHP as a screening tool for possible NCCAH. The recent Endocrine Society guidelines recommend obtaining early morning serum (7:30–8:00 am) 17-OHP levels in symptomatic patients. Morning 17-OHP levels of > 200 ng/dl should prompt further evaluation since it has been shown that levels above 200 ng/dl capture 90% NCCAH individuals [Speiser PW, 2010]. Genetic testing is not considered to be a primary diagnostic tool for NCCAH at this time, but may be helpful in the setting of borderline results or for genetic counseling purposes.

SUMMARY

As most of the investigations are directed to differentiate PCOS/CAH, it is a good principle to remember that high, normal or raised

(150 ng/dl) total testosterone are more likely to be elevated in PCOS than in NCCAH; 70% of patients with PCOS have elevated free testosterone levels, whereas only 44% have elevated total testosterone. Total testosterone levels >150 ng/dl strongly suggest androgen-secreting tumours rather than PCOS or NCCAH. Androstenedione and DHEA may be elevated in either NCCAH or PCOS; in some cases elevation of these secondary androgens are the only indication of hyperandrogenemia. Thus, testing for these two is of a little use.

In essence, the aim of investigations is to isolate the source of androgens. A snapshot view of the salient disorders and their diagnosis is given in Table 3.3. The therapy of these conditions is detailed elsewhere, but this is a sign that acne is a systemic disease and requires clinical and biochemical expertise. Clinicians can pick up cases of PCOS and other hormonal dysfunctions easily in such cases, the treatment of which is gratifying both for the acne but in most cases, helps to enhance the fertility, which is suboptimal in most of these cases.

Table 3.3 *Salient medical disorders that lead to hyperandrogenism*

Systemic disorder	Lab values
Polycystic ovarian syndrome	LH/FSH ratio greater than 2–3 AMH > (6.8 ng/ml)/(3.34 ng/ml) Serum total testosterone 70–120 ng/dL Androstenedione 3–5 ng/ml DHEAS: 50 % of women also have elevation in DHEAS SHBG: Low in 50% of patients with PCOS Prolactin: Mild hyperprolactinaemia 30% of cases
Ovarian tumour	Serum total testosterone greater than 150–200 ng/dl Normal serum DHEAS
Late-onset congenital adrenal hyperplasia	DHEAS 400–800 µg/dl 17-hydroxyprogesterone greater than 200 ng/dL Perform ACTH stimulation test: 17-OH-P > 1000 to 10,000 ng/dl diagnostic of NCCAH
Cushing's syndrome	Overnight dexamethasone suppression test > 5 µg/100 ml
Adrenal tumour	DHEAS > 800 µg/dl Serum total testosterone greater than 150–200 ng/dl

REFERENCES

1. Andersen A. Revised criteria for PCOS in WHO Group II anovulatory infertility—a revival of hypothalamic amenorrhoea? Clin Endocrinol (Oxf). 2014 Sep 26.

2. Bunker CB, Newton JA, Kilbom J et al. Most women with acne have polycystic ovaries. Br J Dermatol 1989; 121: 675–80.

3. Lauritsen MP, Pinborg A, Loft A, Petersen JH, Mikkelsen AL, Bjerge MR, Nyboe. Clin Endocrinol (Oxf). 2015 Apr;82(4):584-91. doi: 10.1111/cen.12621. Epub 2014 Nov 5.

4. McLaughlin B, Barrett P, Finch T et al. Late onset adrenal hyperplasia in a group of Irish females who presented with hirsutism, irregular menses and/or cystic acne. Clin Endocrinol (Oxf) 1990; 32: 57–64.

5. Parahuleva N, Pehlivanov B, Orbecova M, Uchikova E, Ivancheva H [Anti-Müllerian hormone in the major phenotypes of polycystic ovary syndrome]. Akush Ginekol (Sofiia). 2014;53(5):22–7.

6. Peserico A, Angeloni G, Bertoli P et al. Prevalence of polycystic ovaries in women with acne. Arch Dermatol Res 1989; 281: 502–3.

7. Pinola P, Morin-Papunen LC, Bloigu A, Puukka K, Ruokonen A, Järvelin MR, Franks S, Tapanainen JS, Lashen H. Anti-Müllerian hormone: Correlation with testosterone and oligo- or amenorrhoea in female adolescence in a population-based cohort study. Hum Reprod. 2014 Oct 10; 29(10):2317–25.

8. Placzek M, Degitz K, Schmidth H, Plewig G. Acne fulminans in our patient with late onset congenital adrenal hyperplasia. Lancet 1999; 354:739–40.

9. Speiser PW, Azziz R, Baskin LS, et al. Congenital adrenal hyperplasia due to steroid 21-hydroxylase deficiency: An Endocrine Society clinical practice guideline. J Clin Endocrinol Metab. 2010; 95:4133–60. [PubMed: 20823466]

10. Wiweko B, Maidarti M, Priangga MD, Shafira N, Fernando D, Sumapraja K, Natadisastra M, Hestiantoro A. Anti-Müllerian hormone as a diagnostic and prognostic tool for PCOS patients. J Assist Reprod Genet. 2014 Oct;31(10): 1311–6.

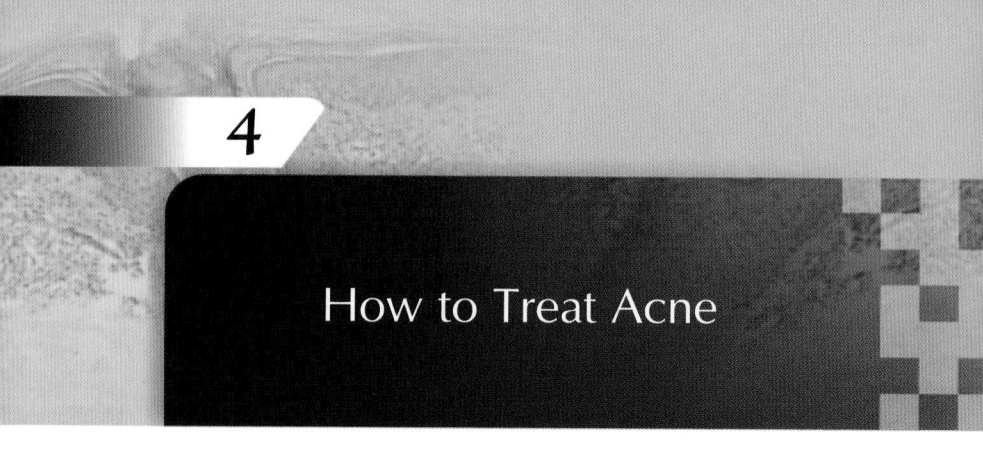

4

How to Treat Acne

I. TOPICAL AGENTS

Acne is a disease caused by inflammation of the pilosebaceous apparatus. It affects more than 85% of teenagers. It typically starts at puberty and resolves slowly around the third decade of life [Ayer J, 2006]. It is usually considered as a benign self-limiting physiological process among adolescent but is better regarded as a disease due to its inflammatory component [Tutakne MA, 2008]. Its implications go far more than its apparent cosmetic nature with severe psychosocial burden in the affected individual. It is important for family physicians to be knowledgeable about the treatment of this common disorder.

The effect on the quality of life has been estimated to be as great as that associated with epilepsy, asthma, diabetes, or arthritis [Mallon EM, 1999].

TOPICAL TREATMENT OF ACNE

The aim of treatment is targeted towards reducing the aetiological factors affecting acne. Depending on the severity of acne, topical medications constitute the sole treatment in many patients with acne and are part of the therapeutic regimen in almost all patients [Russell JJ, 2000].

The nature of the patient's skin has to assessed in order to determine the vehicle to be used (Table 4.1).

Table 4.1 *Various vehicles with respect to the type of skin*		
Dry skin	*Oily skin*	*Sensitive skin*
Creams	Gel	Creams
Lotions	Solutions	Lotions

In oily skin, gels and solution based medication are preferred, which due to its alcohol content which dries the skin. In dry and sensitive skin, gels and solutions are not preferred due to their irritant potential (Table 4.2).

Table 4.2 List of topical agents with their formulations and mode of application [Russell JJ, 2000]		
Agent	**Formulation**	**Method of application**
Benzoyl peroxide	2.5%, 4%, 5%, 10% gels, solutions, face wash and soaps	Once or twice a day
Clindamycin	1% gel	Twice a day
Erythromycin	2% cream	Twice a day
Tretinoin	0.025%, 0.04%, 0.05% and 0.1% gels or creams	Once at night
Adapelene	0.1% gels or solutions	Once at night
Tazarotene	0.05% or 0.1%	Small amount once at night
Salicylic acid	2% gel, 1% or 2% face wash	Once or twice a day
Glycolic acid	6% and 12% creams	Twice a day
Azelaic acid	10% and 20 % cream	Twice a day
Metronidazole	0.75%, 1% gel	Twice a day
Dapsone	5% gel	Twice a day
Sodium sulfacetamide	Sulphur 5%	Twice a day
Precipitated sulphur	5–10% cream	Twice a day
Niacinamide	4 % gel	Twice a day
Nadifloxacin	1% gel	Twice a day

A. Benzoyl Peroxide (BPO)

The main indication of BPO is mild inflammatory (papulopustular) acne as monotherapy, as well as moderate inflammatory acne in combination with other acne treatments. Notably BPO reduces antibiotic-resistant propionibacteria, e.g. induced by topical treatment with antibiotics.

- Broad spectrum bactericidal agent derived from organic peroxides.
- Mechanism of action: Non-specific oxidising activity on *P. acnes*, inhibits triglyceride hydrolysis and reduces inflammation in acne lesions.

- Has comedolytic and keratolytic properties.
- Effective on both inflammatory and non-inflammatory acne.
  In mild acne the effects are visible from 1 to 2 weeks onwards and a 4–8 week course is generally required. Long-term treatment or short contact therapy with a BPO rinse-off product can follow to prevent relapse. A controlled study shows that 2.5% and 5% are equally effective as 10%, the side effects being less [Lassus A, 1981].
- *Combinations*: Benzoyl peroxide combination with clindamycin 1 % and Adapalene 1% is more superior than the drug alone. The improved efficacy of tretinoin 0.05% in combination with benzoyl peroxide (BPO) compared to each of the active ingredient alone has been shown [Handojo I, 1979]. Tretinoin microsphere gel showed improved stability toward UV and oxidative-induced degradation [Shalita AR]. Its combination with a BPO 6% cleanser resulted in a greater reduction of inflammatory acne lesions than monotherapy with 0.1% tretinoin microsphere [Shalita AR, 1989]. The combination of clindamycin and benzoyl peroxide with tretinoin was well tolerated and showed improved efficacy as compared to tretinoin combined with clindamycin; however, the addition of tretinoin to the combination of clindamycin and BPO induced no additional efficacy [Bowman S, 2005]. The efficacy of adapalene gel 0.1% reduces and prevents the development of micro-comedones as recently shown in a 12-week maintenance treatment study after previous combination therapy with BPO 2.5% and adapalene 0.1% in patients with mild to moderate acne [Thielitz A, 2007].
- *Side effects*: Redness, desquamation, and a burning sensation of treated skin are dose-dependent major symptoms of therapy. The most frequent side effect of BPO is skin irritation which is linked to concentration and formulation. High BPO concentrations can exhibit significant irritative effects, especially in alcohol-containing gels. In Indian skin this can cause post-inflammatory hyperpigmentation. Thus a lower concentrations (3–5%) or lower application frequency (e.g. every other day) or a microsphere preparation can help. Rare side effects include sensitization and cause allergic contact dermatitis [Mathaparthi K, 2013].
- *Pregnancy category*: Category C.
- *Keynote*: Benzoyl peroxide has not been associated with bacterial resistance.

B. Topical Antibiotics

The commonly used topical antibiotics used in acne include clindamycin, erythromycin and nadifloxacin. They mainly act on mild to moderate inflammatory acne, with some efficacy in comedones as well. The main problem remains the risk of development of bacterial resistance, which is still under-investigated in acne patients. Thus, the recommendations are to avoid using topical antibiotics alone and for a long duration and to preferentially combine them with benzoyl peroxide or topical retinoids.

1. Clindamycin

- Synthetic broad spectrum antibacterial agent derived from lincomycin, which is isolated from *Streptomyces species.*
- *Mechanism of action*: Inhibition of protein synthesis due to reversibly binding on to the 50s subunit of ribosomal RNA subunit [Mathaparthi K, 2013].
- As a monotherapy, it is more effective in inflammatory acne as compared to non-inflammatory.
- *Combinations*: Clindamycin is combined with Adapalene, tretinoin, benzoyl peroxide, niacinamide, zinc acetate in order to increase its efficacy and decrease resistance.
- *Side effects*: Allergy to clindamycin is rare. Erythema, itching, burning, dryness can be due to the vehicle. Although extremely rare, very few cases of pseudomembranous colitis have been reported due to topical clindamycin.
- *Pregnancy category*: Category B.
- *Keynote*: With increasing resistance to clindamycin monotherapy, combination therapies with clindamycin are preferred.

2. Erythromycin

- Macrolide antibiotic derived from *Streptomyces erythraeus.*
- Mechanism of action: Inhibition of protein synthesis due to reversibly binding on to the 50s subunit of ribosomal RNA subunit [Mathaparthi K, 2013].
- As a monotherapy it is more effective in inflammatory acne as compared to non-inflammatory.
- *Combinations*: Combination with zinc acetate reduces resistance of *P. acnes* to erythromycin.
- *Side effects*: Allergy to erythromycin is rare. Erythema, itching, burning, dryness can be due to the vehicle.
- *Pregnancy category*: Category B.
- *Keynote*: Resistance to a few *P. acnes* species, only a few brands available in Indian market.

3. Nadifloxacin

- Nadifloxacin is a synthetic fluoroquinolone derivative (nadifloxacin) approved for topical use in acne vulgaris and skin infections.

- *Mechanism of action*: Inhibits DNA gyrase that is involved in bacterial DNA synthesis and replication.
- As a monotherapy nadifloxacin 1% cream as efficacious and safe as erythromycin 2% and extremely low numbers of nadifloxacin—resistant microorganisms are detected.
- *Combination*: It is combined with Adapalene 0.1% to increase its efficacy.
- *Keynote*: As exposure of pathogenic bacteria to antibiotics results in drug resistance, it is not desirable to use an important, broad-spectrum antibiotic, which belongs to a class of agents widely used systemically to treat a wide variety of infections, as a topically applied preparation.

4. Metronidazole

- Synthetic nitroimidazole which predominantly works on anaerobic organisms.
- *Mechanism of action*: Disruption of DNA and inhibition of nucleic acid synthesis, anti-inflammatory effect include suppression of cell-mediated immunity and leukocyte chemotaxis [Mathaparthi K, 2013].
- As monotherapy, role is unclear in acne vulgaris but effective in acne rosacea.
- *Combinations*: Combination with benzoyl peroxide is more effective than benzoyl peroxide alone.
- *Side effects*: Rare include dryness, itching, burning and stinging.
- *Pregnancy category*: Category B.
- *Keynote*: The drug has no action on *P. acnes*, its effect on acne lesions is probably due to its anti-inflammatory effects.

C. Retinoids

Topical retinoids form an important group in the treatment of acne. The retinoids used in acne therapy are tretinoin, adapalene and tazarotene.

When prescribing a topical retinoid, the following points should be considered for patient counselling:

- Direct and prolonged sun (or artificial UV) exposure should be avoided, and non-comedogenic sunscreens are recommended during the sunny season.
- Excessive washing with soaps should be avoided, and washing should be performed with warm water and a gentle cleanser.
- The retinoid should not be applied directly after shaving, and aggressive astringents or ethanol-containing aftershaves or toners should be avoided.

- The patient should stop all other OTC acne treatments, such as abrasive peelings, except those recommended by the physician.
- Weather extremes such as cold or heat/humidity can worsen the symptoms of retinoid dermatitis. Thus they can be avoided in this season.
- When applying the retinoid to the face, the corners of the eyes and mouth should be avoided, because they are easily irritated.
- The use of a moisturizer for the skin and lipsticks or petrolatum can prevent and alleviate symptoms of retinoid-dermatitis.
- The patient should know that irritation generally occurs in the early treatment phase and reactions often completely disappear upon treatment continuation.
- The time course of the expected improvement should be discussed. The value of treatment should not be judged before 8–12 weeks. However, with the new fixed combination therapies, often a rapid improvement can be seen already after 1 to 2 weeks.

1. Tretinoin

- First naturally occurring retinoid available in the treatment of acne.
- *Mechanism of action*: Topically applied all-trans retinoic acid(tretinoin) is taken up by the keratinocyte, where it binds the cytosolic retinol-binding protein. This complex binds to the nuclear retinoic acid receptors (RAR). This acts as a transcription factor which later binds to the retinoic acid response elements in DNA to induce gene transcription (Sami N, 2013).
- This gene transcription affects the differentiation of cells in the skin and normalises epithelial keratinization.
- As a montherapy in acne it acts on the follicular retention hyperkeratosis and decreases inflammation, therefore, it is useful in all forms of acne.
- *Application of tretinoin*: Since it is photolabile and as it can induce photosensitivity it should be applied at night in minimum quantity. Retinoid dermatitis is usually seen in the first two weeks of therapy which gradually resolves over a period of time. In order to decrease it, retinoids are applied for a short duration (30–60 min) and later washed or applied alternate day.
- *Combinations*:
  Tretinoin-combination therapy—the treatment efficacy of tretinoin can be enhanced by combination with topical antimicrobials. A superiority toward monotherapy has been shown in clinical studies for the combination of tretinoin and erythromycin and with highest evidence levels, for the combination of clindamycin and tretinoin.

The combination with benzoyl peroxide is possible when both substances are applied alternately, e.g. tretinoin in the morning and benzoyl peroxide (BPO) in the evening, to avoid oxidative degradation of tretinoin. The combination of tretinoin microsphere gel combination with a benzoyl peroxide 6% cleanser resulted in a greater reduction of inflammatory acne lesions than the monotherapy with 0.1% tretinoin microsphere, without increased skin irritation.

The efficacy and safety of combination with a fixed clindamycin/BPO preparations has been demonstrated for tretinoin microsphere gel 0.04 and 0.1%. The triple combination showed improved efficacy compared to a combination of tretinoin microsphere and clindamycin, but was comparable to a fixed clindamycin/BPO combination.

- *Side effects*: Temporary worsening of acne, peeling, irritation, erythema, photosensitivity.
- *Pregnancy*: Category C.
- *Keynote*: In addition to its beneficial effect on acne, it is also useful in other dermatological conditions like fine wrinkling, mottled pigmentation, melasma, early stretch marks, prior to certain procedures.

2. *Adapalene*

- A synthetic retinoid which is more photostable and lipophilic than tretinoin.
- *Mechanism of action*: It has a selective affinity for retinoic acid receptors (RAR-β and RAR-γ), thereby reduction the irritant effects seen by tretinoin which binds to all three forms of RARs. It also inhibits chemotaxis of polymorphonuclear leukocytes and release of free oxygen radicals from neutrophils. The lipophilicity accounts for its selective uptake by hair follicle associated sebaceous gland and therefore for its application in acne [Sami N, 2013].
- *Method of application* is similar to tretinoin but less irritant than tretinoin.

A meta-analysis of five well-controlled trials [Cunliffe WJ, 1998] involving more than 900 patients demonstrated equivalent efficacy of adapalene 0.1% and tretinoin 0.025% with a mean reduction of total acne lesions of 57% in patients receiving adapalene for 12 weeks and 53% in those receiving tretinoin, however, with a more rapid onset of action and a considerably greater local tolerability during adapalene treatment. Adapalene gel 0.3% demonstrated superiority to adapalene gel 0.1% and vehicle and was well tolerated.

- *Combinations*: Adapalene is the first topical retinoid whose chemicophysical properties allow a fixed combination with benzoyl peroxide in a stable galenic formulation, which was demonstrated in a multicenter 12-week parallel group study involving 517 subjects with moderate to moderately severe acne. The fixed combination of adapalene 0.1% and benzoyl peroxide 2.5% gel provided significantly greater efficacy for the treatment of acne vulgaris relative to the monotherapies as early as week 1, with a comparable safety profile to adapalene [Thiboutot DM]. Notably adverse events were more frequent with the combination therapy (mainly due to an increase in mild-to-moderate dry skin), occurred early in the study, and were transient.The efficacy of adapalene has also been investigated in combination with a fixed combination of benzoyl peroxide 5 % and clindamycin 1% (BP/C) [Del Rosso JQ, 2007].
- *Side effects*: Peeling, irritation, erythema, photosensitivity.
- *Pregnancy*: Category C.
- *Keynote*: It is better tolerated than tretinoin.

3. Tazarotene

- Synthetic retinoid which rapidly hydrolyses in tissue to active metabolite tazarotenic acid.
- *Mechanism of action*: It has affinity for all three RARs but more on RAR-γ. It blocks ornithine decarboxylase activity with decreased cell proliferation and hyperplasia, therefore resulting in keratolytic and comedolytic activity in acne [Sami N, 2013].
- *Method of application*: Similar to tretinoin.
- *Side effects*: Irritation, erythema, burning, pruritus, photosensitivity, dry skin and teratogenic potential.
- *Pregnancy*: Absolute contraindication (X).
- *Keynote*: Its use in acne is restricted due to its irritant potential.

D. Miscellaneous Agents

1. Salicylic Acid

- One of the oldest known topical medications in dermatology derived from willow bark and wintergreen leaves.
  Although various concentrations exist (0.5–10%), 2% is the maximum strength allowed by the FDA in OTC products.
- *Mechanism of action*: It is lipid soluble molecule which is miscible with lipids present on the superficial epidermis and sebaceous gland of the hair follicle. Therefore, it causes loosening and detachment of keratinocytes. It is believed to have a comedolytic action also. It also possesses an anti-inflammatory action.

- It is usually used in combination with other therapeutic modalities in acne. It is effective in non-inflammatory dermatoses.

  A 12-week study found 2% SA cream superior to 5% BPO cream in reducing closed comedones, 2 open comedones, inflammatory lesions, and total lesions [Zander E, 1992]. A 4-week crossover study comparing a 2% SA acne cleanser to a 10% BPO wash demonstrated that only patients treated with the SA cleanser had a significant decrease in comedonal lesions [Shalita AR, 1989]. Stated differently, both groups demonstrated significant improvement in comedonal count when treated with SA, whereas BPO treatment either worsened or insignificantly improved comedonal quantity. Recently, a small study comparing a 2% SA/1% clindamycin combination with placebo demonstrated a significant reduction in inflammatory and non-inflammatory lesions, with 71% of subjects reporting improvement after 8 weeks (compared to 11% of placebo group) [Touitou E, 2008].

- *Side effects*: Systemic effects (salicylism) is rare when used for acne. Other side effects are irritation, erythema.
- *Pregnancy*: To be avoided during pregnancy.
- *Keynote*: It is one of the better therapeutic options in patients with oily skin.

2. Glycolic Acid

- It is an α-hydroxy acid which are carboxylic acids with a hydroxyl group on the adjacent carbon. It is a two-carbon molecule with a formula $HOCH_2COOH$.
- *Mechanism of action*: It induces a localised decrease in calcium ion concentration in epidermis which leads to desquamation and retards differentiation of keratinocytes. Long-term application has benefits on the dermal collagen, elastin and glycosaminoglycans.
- It can be used in both inflammatory and non-inflammatory acne. Both 6% and 12% can be used as "office peels".
- As a combination it is given along with topical retinoids.
- *Side effects*: Irritation, dermatitis, pigmentary disturbances, photosensitivity can occur.
- *Pregnancy*: Category B.
- *Keynote*: It is also used as a chemical peel for facial melanosis, aging of skin.

3. Azelaic Acid

Azelaic acid is a C-9 dicarboxylic acid.

- It is a naturally occurring dicarboxylic acid bactericidal against *P. acnes* [Mathaparthi K, 2013].

- *Mechanism of action*: Disruption of mitochondrial respiration and protein synthesis, inhibits division and differentiation of keratinocytes. The diacid reduces *Propionibacterium acnes* proliferation. It interferes with sebogenesis and possesses anti-inflammatory activity.
- As a monotherapy it is effective in inflammatory and non-inflammatory acne.
- *Combinations*: Efficacy of azelaic acid combination with erythromycin is more effective than drug alone.
- *Side effects*: Local irritation, redness is common in the first two weeks of application which gradually subsides.
- *Pregnancy category*: Category B.
- *Keynote*: Gel based preparation are more effective than cream but they are preferably avoided in sensitive skin.

4. Dapsone

- Synthetic sulfone which has antimicrobial and anti-inflammatory action on *M. leprae*.
- *Mechanism of action*: Inhibits bacterial dihydropteroate synthetase, an enzyme affecting folic acid synthesis [Mathaparthi K, 2013].
- As a monotherapy it is effective in inflammatory and non-inflammatory acne.
- No combination are available.
- *Side effects*: Erythema, dryness or sunburn.
- *Pregnancy*: Category C.
- *Keynote*: Dapsone gel has recently been made available in the Indian market.

5. Sodium Sulfacetamide

- Aniline derivative which acts on *P. acnes*.
- *Mechanism of action*: Inhibits bacterial dihydropteroate synthetase, an enzyme affecting folic acid synthesis [Mathaparthi K, 2013].
- In combination with sulphur, a nonspecific antifungal and antibacterial it is effective in treatment of acne.
- *Pregnancy*: Category C.
- *Keynote*: Presently unavailable in the Indian market.

6. Sulphur

- Used in medicine since biblical times.
- The most common form used in dermatology is precipitated sulphur. It is produced by adding sublimed sulphur with lime, water and hydrochloric acid.

- *Mechanism of action*: It is believed to have antiseptic, antiparasitic, antiacne, and antiseborrheic properties. It binds with cysteine in the keratinocytes to induce keratolytic action [Mathaparthi K, 2013].
- It is combined with sulfacetamide has a synergistic effect in acne as it is keratolytic and sulfacetamide is an antibacterial agent.
- *Pregnancy category*: Though there are no well-defined studies on its effects in pregnancy, sulphur has been used in treatment of scabies in pregnancy before the advent of permethrin.
- *Keynote*: A few brands of precipitated sulphur available in the Indian market.

7. Niacinamide

- Nicotinic acid (vitamin B_3) is an essential vitamin which is converted in the body to niacinamide.
- Coenzyme in many oxidation-reduction reactions.
- *Mechanism of action*: It mainly inhibits lysosomal enzyme release, inhibits lymphocytic transformation and stabilises leukocytes.
- In acne it is mainly used as an adjunctive therapy along with clindamycin.
- *Side effects*: Due to effects of the gel base like irritation, erythema.
- *Keynote*: It also stabilises epidermal barrier function, increases keratinocyte differentiation, therefore, used as topical therapy for aging.

FIXED DOSE COMBINATIONS (FDC) IN ACNE

Since the mechanism of action of each agent used in acne was limited, different agents (creams) had to be used in the treatment to increase the overall efficacy, thereby increasing the complexity of treatment regimen. In order to overcome this deficiency, a concept of fixed dose combinations was introduced (Table 4.3) [Del Rosso JQ, 2009].

The advantages of FDC are:
- Enhancing compliance by simplifying treatment regimen
- Improving efficacy and tolerability
- Addressing many of the aetiological factors

The various FDC available are:
- Tretinoin 0.025% and clindamycin 1%
- Adapalene 0.1% and clindamycin 1%
- Benzoyl peroxide 2.5%/5% and clindamycin 1%
- Benzoyl peroxide 2.5% and Adapalene 0.1%
- Benzoyl peroxide 10% and precipitated sulphur 5%
- Clindamycin 1% and niacinamide 4%

FDC	Hyperkeratosis	P. acnes	Sebum	Inflammation	Tolerability
Table 4.3: *Efficacy and Tolerability of FDC*					
Tretinoin 0.025% and clindamycin 1%	+++	+++	++	++	Irritant potential present
Adapalene 0.1% and clindamycin 1%	+++	+++	++	++	Less as compared to tretinoin
Benzoyl peroxide 2.5%/5% and clindamycin 1%	+	+++	+	+	Irritant potential
Benzoyl peroxide 2.5% and adapelene 0.1%	+++	+++	++	++	Irritant potential
Benzoyl peroxide 10% and precipitated sulphur 5%	++	+++	++	+	Irritant potential
Clindamycin 1% and niacinamide 4%		+++	+	+	Better tolerability

REFERENCES

1. Ayer J, Burrows N. Acne: More than skin deep. Postgrad Med J 2006; 82:500–506.

2. Bowman S, Gold M, Nasir A, et al. Comparison of clindamycin/benzoyl peroxide, tretinoin plus clindamycin, and the combination of clindamycin/benzoyl peroxide and tretinoin plus clindamycin in the treatment of acne vulgaris: a randomized, blinded study. J Drugs Dermatol. 2005; 4:611–8.

3. Cunliffe WJ, Poncet M, Loesche C, Verschoore M. A comparison of the efficacy and tolerability of adapalene 0.1% gel versus tretinoin 0.025% gel in patients with acne vulgaris: a meta-analysis of five randomized trials. Br J Dermatol. 1998; 139 Suppl 52:48–56.

4. Del Rosso JQ. Study results of benzoyl peroxide 5%/clindamycin 1% topical gel, adapalene 0.1% gel, and use in combination for acne vulgaris. J Drugs Dermatol. 2007; 6 (6):616–22.

5. Del Rosso JQ. The role of fixed-dose combination topical therapy in the treatment of acne vulgaris. The dermatologist 2009; 17. retrieved on march 4, 2015 from http//www.the-dermatologist.com/content/the-role-fixed-dose-combination-topical-therapy-treatment-acne-vulgaris.htm.

6. Handojo I. Retinoic acid cream (Airol cream) and benzoyl-peroxide in the treatment of acne vulgaris. Southeast Asian J Trop Med Public Health. 1979; 10:548–51.

7. Holland KT, Bojar RA, Cunliffe WJ, Cutcliffe AG, et al. The effect of zinc and erythromycin on the growth of erythromycin-resistant and erythromycin- sensitive isolates of Propionibacterium acnes: an in- vitro study. Br J Dermatol. 1992; 126:505–9.

8. Lassus A. Local treatment of acne. A clinical study and evaluation of the effect of different concentrations of benzoyl peroxide gel. Curr Med Res Opin. 1981; 7:370–3.

9. Mallon EM, Newton JN, Klassen A, et al. The quality of life in acne: a comparison with general medical conditions using generic questionnaires. Br J Dermatol 1999; 140:672–6

10. Mathaparthi K, Hsu S. Topical antibacterial agents. In: Wolverton SE, comprehensive dermatologic drug therapy. 3rd edition. Elsevier India; 2013.p. 452–459.

11. Russell J.J. Topical Therapy for Acne. Am Fam Physician. 2000; 61:357–365.

12. Sami N. Topical retinoids. In Wolverton SE, comprehensive dermatologic drug therapy. 3rd edition. Elsevier India; 2013. p. 505–517

13. Shalita AR, Rafal ES, Anderson DN, et al. Compared ef? cacy and safety of tretinoin 0.1% microsphere gel alone and in combination with benzoyl peroxide 6% cleanser for the treatment of acne vulgaris. Cutis. 2003; 72:167–72.

14. Shalita AR. Comparison of a salicylic acid cleanser and a benzoyl peroxide wash in the treatment of acne vulgaris. Clin Ther. 1989; 11(2):264–7.

15. Thiboutot DM, Weiss J, Bucko A, Eichenfield L, Jones T, Clark S, et al. Adapalene-benzoyl peroxide, a fixed-dose combination for the treatment of acne vulgaris: Results of a multicenter, randomized double- blind, controlled study. J Am Acad Dermatol. 2007; 57:791–9.

16. Thielitz A, Sidou F, Gollniick H. Control of micro-comedone formation throughout a maintenance treatment with adapalene gel, 0.1%. J Eur Acad Dermatol Venereol. 2007; 21:747–53.

17. Touitou E, et al. Efficacy and tolerability of clindamycin phosphate and salicylic acid gel in the treatment of mild to moderate acne vulgaris. J Eur Acad Dermatol Venereol. 2008; 22(5):629–31.

18. Tutakne MA, Vaishampayan SS. Acne, rosacea and perioral dermatitis. InValia RG, Valia AR, editors. IADVL textbook of dermatology. 3rd ed. Mumbai: Bhalani publishing house; 2008. p. 837–854.

19. Zander E, Weisman S. Treatment of acne vulgaris with salicylic acid pads. Clin Ther. 1992; 14(2):247–53.

II. NOVEL DRUG DELIVERY STRATEGIES AND ACNE VULGARIS

SKIN AS A SITE FOR DRUG DELIVERY

The skin has historically been used for the topical delivery of compounds, it is only since the 1970s with the advent of transdermal patches that it has widely been used as a route for systemic delivery [SD Roy, et al, 1996].

Nanoparticle delivery to the skin is being increasingly used to facilitate local therapies. The nanoparticle definition designated by the National Nanotechnology Initiative has been adopted by the American National Standards Institute as particles with all dimensions between 1 nm and 100 nm [FAQ]. Figure 4.1 shows that the potential sites for targeting nanoparticles include the surface of the skin, furrows and hair follicles. A recent review by Baroli discusses nanoparticle penetration largely from the skin structure perspective. The title of this review *Penetration of Nanoparticles and Nanomaterials in the Skin: Fiction or Reality?* highlights the ongoing debate of nanoparticle penetration

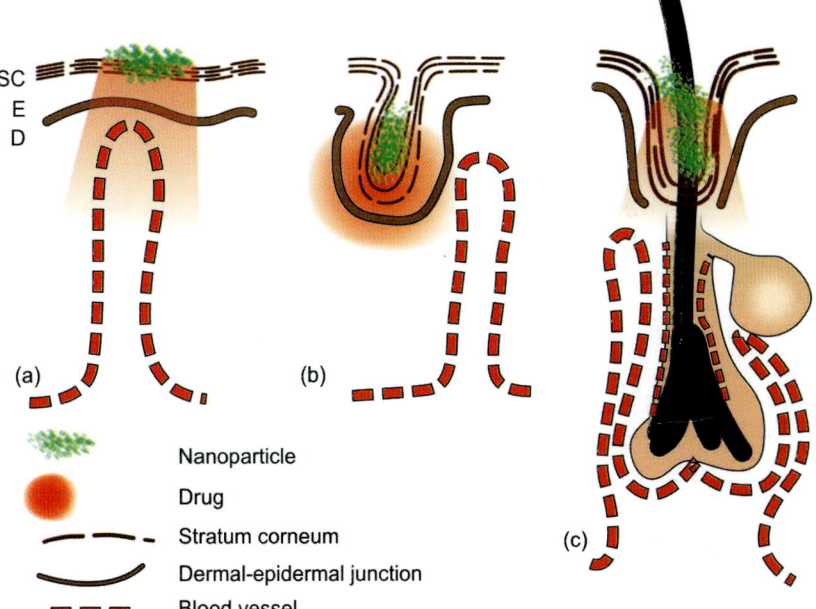

Fig. 4.1: Sites in skin for nanoparticle delivery. Topical nanoparticle drug delivery takes place in three major sites: stratum corneum **[SC]** surface (a), furrows (dermatoglyphs) (b), and openings of hair follicles (infundibulum) (c). The nanoparticles are shown in green and the drug in red. Other sites for delivery are the viable epidermis **[E]** and dermis **[D]**

[Baroli B, 2010]. This debate is fuelled by the need for more rigorous, multidisciplinary approaches to shed light on mechanisms of particle penetration and interactions with skin. Likewise, Schneider et al. (2009) make a compelling case in their review on nanoparticle skin interactions for more rigorous studies on the effects of hydration and mechanical stress on skin with regard to nanoparticle–skin interactions.

Particles can interact with skin at a cellular level as adjuvants. This nanoparticle–skin interaction can be used to enhance immune reactivity for topical vaccine applications. Another example of nanoparticle–skin interactions is the topical use of silver nanoparticles as over the counter antimicrobial agents [J Tian, 2007], where the nanoparticles provide a slow release of silver ions that have wound healing and antimicrobial properties. The silver ions released from nanoparticle can inhibit microbial proliferation, but also accelerate wound healing. This controlled release of silver ions while the nanoparticles remain on the skin surface highlights one of the most successful topical nanoparticle drug delivery strategies.

Generally, the promise of nanoparticle-mediated drug delivery into the epidermis and dermis without barrier modification has met with a little success. Where the barrier is compromised, however, such as in aged or diseased skin, there may be potential for enhanced particle penetration. Ulcerated squamous cell carcinoma is one example. The opportunities and obstacles for nanoparticle drug delivery are only just beginning to be explored in ongoing clinical trials. For instance, capsaicin-loaded nanoparticles are being used to treat the pain associated with diabetic neuropathy. Advances in particle engineering, formulation science and an improved understanding of nanoparticle–skin interactions will undoubtedly lead to important clinically relevant improvements in topical drug delivery. An overriding concern is the safety of any applied nanoparticle, recognising the possibility that non-biodegradable nanoparticles could be taken up and retained by the reticuloendothelial system [S. Erdogan, 2009]. In addition, there is the potential for local toxicity, shown by a recent report of nanoparticles inducing keratinocyte apoptosis, where the subtle relationship between longer and shorter phosphatidylcholine chain lengths makes the difference between life and death for keratinocytes [CH Liang, 2009]. This illustrates the need for toxicity monitoring *in vitro* and especially *in vivo*.

DRUG CARRIER SYSTEMS USED IN PILOSEBACEOUS TARGETING

The goal of using a drug delivery system is to convey a sufficient dose of a drug to a specific site. It is well recognized that for certain drug delivery systems, hair follicles are privileged penetration pathways. They enter faster into these shunts than through the stratum corneum and hereby offer the possibility to create high local concentrations of the active compounds within the follicular duct.

In recent years, many attempts have been made to enhance drug deposition in the PSU using delivery systems such as nanoemulsions, solid lipid nanoparticles, low-molecular weight dextrans, microspheres iontophoresis and niosomes or liposomes. Among the various drug delivery systems, which are currently under investigation for topical therapy, *liposomes*, and *microspheres* are most widely used. Micro- as well as nanoparticles have also been demonstrated to reach deep into the hair follicles, where the barrier possesses only a few layers of differentiated corneocytes and can be considered highly permeable, and additionally the hair follicles can act as long-term reservoir, beneficial condition when transdermal delivery is intended.

1. Pilosebaceous Targeting by Liposomes

Mezei and Gulasekharam in 1980 identified the potential of liposomes (Fig. 4.2) for topical therapy which leads to further investigation and development of lipid vesicles as carriers for skin delivery of drugs. Conflicting results continued to be published concerning their effectiveness, enhancing the controversy of liposome as dermal and

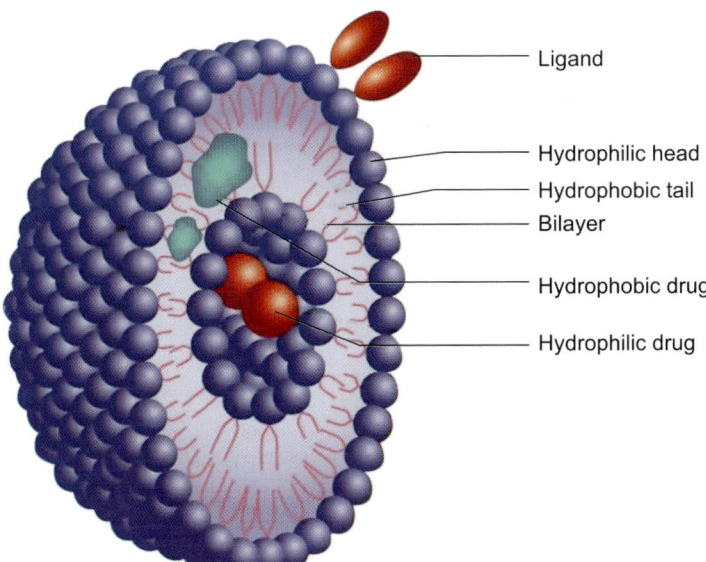

Ligand

Hydrophilic head
Hydrophobic tail
Bilayer

Hydrophobic drug

Hydrophilic drug

Fig. 4.2: Liposome and its different drug-loading and surface functionalization modalities

transdermal drug delivery vehicles. The first therapeutic liposomes containing the anti-mycotic agent, econazole, were commercialized shortly before the year 1990. Among the chemical enhancers such as oils, surfactants and solvents used to increase trasnsdermal delivery; liposomes have the advantage in overcoming the lipoidal environment of the hair follicle because of the 'wetting' phenomena of the liposome itself and its ability to penetrate the follicle cell membrane. Thus, liposomes have been widely used to enhance transfollicular and transdermal delivery of the low/high molecular weight hydrophilic/lipophilic compounds.

2. Pilosebaceous Targeting by Niosomes

Non-ionic surfactant based vesicles (niosomes) are formed from the self-assembly of non-ionic amphiphiles in aqueous media resulting in closed bilayer structures (Fig. 4.3). The assembly into closed bilayers is rarely spontaneous and usually involves some input of energy such as physical agitation or heat. The result is an assembly in which the hydrophobic parts of the molecule are shielded from the aqueous solvent and the hydrophilic head groups enjoy maximum contact with the same. These structures are analogous to phospholipid vesicles (liposomes) and are able to encapsulate aqueous solutes and serve as drug carriers. The low cost, greater stability and ease of storage of non-ionic surfactants has presented these vesicles as an alternative to phospholipids.

Non-ionic surfactants overwhelm the problem of natural variability of phospholipids and are reported to follow the pilosebaceous route for entry into systemic circulation when vesicles based on these surfactants are applied topically. Niosomes formation involves a particular class of amphiphiles and aqueous solvent. In some cases, cholesterol is required for vesicle formation and vesicle aggregation may be overcome by inclusion of molecules that stabilize the system against the formation of aggregates by repulsive steric or electrostatic effects.

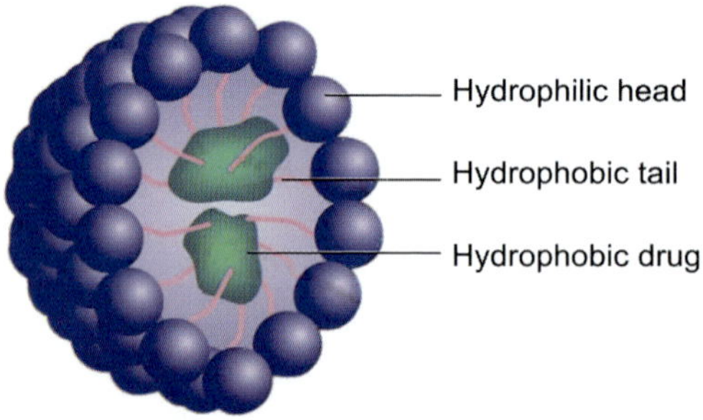

Hydrophilic head

Hydrophobic tail

Hydrophobic drug

Fig. 4.3: Niosome and its internal synthetic surfactant surrounding drug payload

Appreciable deposition of 3 H-cimetidine was attained into the pilosebaceous unit of the hamster ear after topical application of 50% ethanol solution (pH 7.4), glyceryl-dilaurate-based non-ionic liposomes (pH 5.5) and egg phosphatidylcholine-based liposomes (pH 5.5). It has been shown that hydroalcoholic and non-ionic liposome solutions appeared equipotent in suppressing sebaceous gland growth, whereas phospholipid liposomes had almost no pharmacological effect. The reason behind the inactivity of the phospholipid liposome formulation was explained as being an ion-pairing phenomenon at the pH of the formulation. These interesting results made the formulation factors, particularly charge effects, as influenced by pH, an important concern.

Advantages of liposomes and niosomes over conventional non-vesicle formulations.

Their amphipathic nature, which allows incorporation of a wide variety of hydrophilic and hydrophobic drugs.

- They may serve as a solubilizing matrix.
- As local depot for sustained release.
- As permeation enhancers of dermally active compounds.
- As a rate limiting membrane for the modulation of systemic absorption of drugs via the skin.

3. Pilosebaceous Targeting by Microspheres

The microspheres are characteristically free flowing powders consisting of proteins or synthetic polymers, which are biodegradable in nature, and ideally having a particle size less than 200 μm (Fig. 4.4). Microspheres are very stable, easy to couple with other molecules,

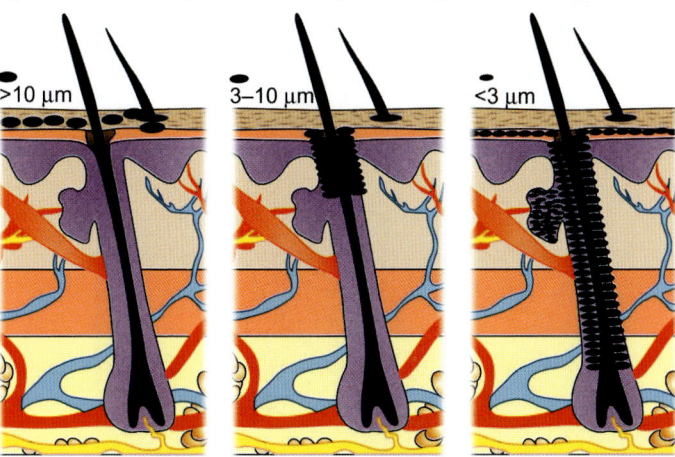

Fig. 4.4: Ideal size parameters that determine penetration into the pilosebaceous unit

easy to prepare or purchase in different well-defined sizes and are well documented in both *in-vivo* and *in-vitro* investigations. Advantages of microspheres for follicular targeting:

- Good stability on application in the skin.
- Easy penetration with a defined mean size in a narrow size distribution.
- Protection of the drug against degradation in the formulation (oxidation, hydrolysis) or premature inactivation on the skin surface.
- Controlled release of the drug in the hair follicles.
- Possibility of incorporating either lipophilic or hydrophilic drugs.
- Site specific targeting, for example, to the pilosebaceous structures.

The size of microspheres has been shown to have a major influence on follicular targeting. Earlier studies as done on size-characterized fluorescent polystyrene microspheres in suspension showed that the propensity of the microspheres to penetrate the skin appendages is proportional to their size [Schaefer H, 1990] (Fig. 4.2). Larger microspheres (>10 µm) neither penetrate into the follicular orifices nor the horny layer, whereas the 9 and 10 µm beads concentrate around the opening the follicles without further penetration. 7 µm microspheres are frequently observed deep in the follicular canal but rarely penetrate the SC. Depending on the microsphere size, microspheres of 5 µm show a high concentration in the follicular ducts, but without penetrating through the SC (Fig. 4.5).

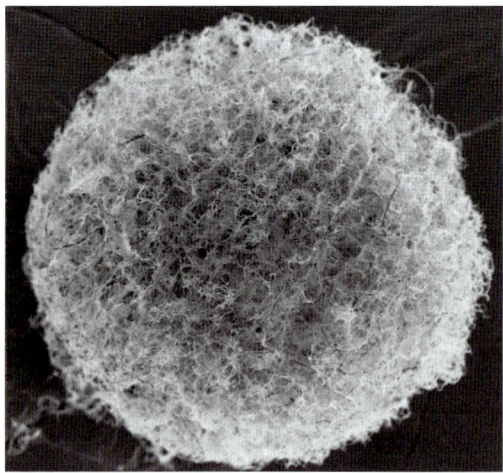

Fig. 4.5: A microsphere of a size of 50 µm. Each cavity of the microsphere contains the active which permeates the pilosebaceous unit to act on the target site. Ideal penetration size <5 µm

4. Pilosebaceous Targeting by Nanoemulsions

Nanoemulsions are transparent, liquid isotropic dispersions composed of water, oil and surfactants and are thermodynamically stable [Osborne DW, 1988] of a size of 50 to 200 nm. At precise compositions of the ingredients their formation is spontaneous and high shear energies are not required for their preparation, essentially reducing the likelihood of protein or plasmid DNA degradation during formulation processing. Since they are thermodynamically stable, they can be prepared with low shear methods and are capable of encapsulating defined amounts of water.

Water-in-oil nanoemulsions have been reported to improve absorption of water-soluble peptides following intraduodenal administration. There are relatively fewer studies that address the feasibility of topical delivery from nanoemulsions. Although nanoemulsions possess several advantages with regard to their ease of preparation, high stability and clarity, the most commonly examined systems include short-chain alcohols such as butanol, pentanol and hexanol as well as non-polar phases such as hexane that make them unsuitable for pharmaceutical purposes. Thus, it would be desirable to use nanoemulsions that can be prepared on a large scale with oils and surfactants that are safe, non-toxic, non-irritating and with components that are generally regarded as safe (GRAS). Advantages offered by nanoemulsions for follicular targeting are:

1. Poorly soluble drugs could be easily formulated.
2. Increases the skin permeation rate and enhance the topical effect due to prolonged residence time in the uppermost skin layers due to the large surface area and low surface tension of the oil droplets.
3. Formation is spontaneous and high shear energies are not required for their preparation and hence enabling formulation of proteins and plasmid DNA.
4. High thermodynamic stability

5. Pilosebaceous Targeting by Nanoparticles

Nanoparticles are subnanosized colloidal structures composed of synthetic or semi-synthetic polymers. Over the past 15 years, polymeric nanocapsules and nanospheres have been extensively studied as drug carriers in the pharmaceutical field as well as an efficient coating material to control the drug release from microparticles [Beck RCR, 2007]. Nanospheres are defined as a matricial polymeric structure, in which drugs can be entrapped or molecularly dispersed. On the other hand, nanocapsules are characterized by a lipophilic core surrounded by a polymeric layer, in which drugs can be dissolved in the oil, dispersed within the particle or adsorbed at the interface particle/ water.

Skin penetration of polymeric nanoparticles has been investigated less than that of liposomes and solid lipid nanoparticles. When these systems are applied epicutaneously, they can alter the drug pharmacokinetic and biodistribution through skin. Besides, their small size facilitates their formulation in dermatological products and enables comfortable application to the skin [Guterres SS, 2007]. Follicular penetration of nanoparticles appears to be a promising mechanism for drug delivery.

6. Pilosebaceous Targeting by Lipid Nanocarriers

Both solid lipid nanoparticles (SLN) and nanostructured lipid carriers (NLC) have been introduced as an alternative carrier system to traditional carriers, such as emulsions, liposomes, polymeric nanoparticles for pharmaceutical drugs and cosmetic active ingredients. Both, SLN and NLC, are composed of physiological and biodegradable lipids, which possess a low cytotoxicity and also low systemic toxicity. SLN consists of pure solid lipid while NLC are made of a solid matrix entrapping liquid lipid compartment. Solid lipid nanoparticles are submicron colloidal carriers (50–1000 nm) which are composed of physiological lipid, dispersed in water or in an aqueous surfactant solution. SLN as colloidal carriers combines the advantages of polymeric nanoparticles, fat emulsions and liposomes simultaneously and avoiding some of their disadvantages. In order to overcome the disadvantages associated with the liquid state of the oil droplets, the liquid lipid was replaced by a solid lipid, which eventually transformed into solid lipid nanoparticles.

VARIOUS NOVEL DRUG DELIVERY STRATEGIES IN ACNE VULGARIS

In case of dermatological pharmacotherapy, for the treatment of skin inflammatory and infectious disorders like acne, the dermal delivery of active ingredients is desirable. Topical application of antiacne agents assures many advantages over oral or intravenous administration such as it offers avoidance of first pass metabolism and elimination of gastrointestinal irritation (Table 4.4). Skin being an effective barrier for foreign permeation encumbers the access of antiacne agents to the pathologic site, thereby decreasing its bioavailability. Therefore, the topical dosage forms against acne should be designed such that topical dosage form facilitates the delivery of active moiety to the target site that is pilosebaceous unit of the skin. With this intention, an intelligently framed delivery system encapsulating the active moiety

Table 4.4 *Overview of novel topical delivery system in acne*

Novel drug delivery carrier	Drug entrapped	Method of preparation	Problem statement	Advantages
Nanoparticles	Chitosan alginate Minocycline	Ultrasonication Ion pairing	Low solubility	Enhanced antimicrobial activity
			Lack of drug loading and entrapment efficiency due to hydrophilicity of the drug	Enhanced drug loading and entrapment efficiency controlled release
	Azelaic acid	Emulsification solvent diffusion	Fewer side effects	Enhanced drug retention at PSU and stability
	Triclosan	Solvent displacement	Insufficient permeation and absorption via cutaneous route	Non-irritant to skin, enhanced stability
	Cyproterone acetate	Ultrasonication	Systemic antiandrogenic effects	Increased skin penetration and absorption
	Garcinia mangostana	Solvent displacement Ion gelation reaction	Water insolubility	Increased follicular penetration and absorption; increased therapeutic activity
	Gallidermin	Freeze drying	For oral administration only and systemic pass demerits	Topical formulation with enhanced chemical stability
Niosomes	Tretinoin	Thin film hydration	Photodegradation	Increased accumulation in superficial stratum and stability. Increased drug

Contd.

Table 4.4 *Overview of novel topical delivery system in acne (Contd.)*

Novel drug delivery carrier	Drug entrapped	Method of preparation	Problem statement	Advantages
				release and entrapment efficiencies
	Rosmarinic acid	Reverse phase evaporation	Low water solubility	Increased skin retention of drug and facilitated prolong release
	Isotretinoin	Sonication	Skin irritation, very low water solubility, difficulty to incorporate in topical base, photodegradation	Potential for skin targeting, prolonging drug release, reduction of photodegradation and skin irritation
	Clindamycin hydrochloride	Film formation	Lesser reduction in number of lesions	Enhanced antiacne activity and sustained release of drug
	Finasteride	Film formation	Only oral administration possible	Topical application with enhanced drug concentration
Liposomes	Tretinoin	Film formation	Skin irritant, photo instability	Enhanced local tolerability and 5–6 times increase comedolytic activity. Reduced photo instability
	Tea tree oil	Ultrasonication	Lesser absorption via follicular route	Facilitated follicular route absorption
	Salicylic acid	Thin film hydration	Skin irritant	Increased entrapment efficiency and stability

Contd.

Table 4.4 Overview of novel topical delivery system in acne (Contd.)

Novel drug delivery carrier	Drug entrapped	Method of preparation	Problem statement	Advantages
	Cyproterone acetate	-	Systemic antiandrogenic effects	Increased activity by reducing acne lesions and adverse effects
	Benzoyl peroxide	Film hydration	Skin irritation	Improved antibacterial activity, reduced irritation
Solid nanoparticles	Isotretinoin	Microemulsification	Teratogenicity, mucocutaneous problems like cheilitis, dermatitis, conjunctivitis, blepharitis, skin fragility and xerosis, psychological disorders, erythema, dryness, itching, stinging, skin peeling	Reduced dermal irritation, increased therapeutic performance
	Retinoic acid	Hot melt homogenization	Sensitive to sunlight, eczematous irritation, erythema, interaction with other applied products	Comedolytic effect, reduction in RA induced irritation
	Neem oil	Double emulsification	Lesser drug absorption	Prolonged treatment of acne
	Tretinoin	Hot high pressure homogenization	Skin irritation and chemical instability	High encapsulation efficacy, physical stability and absence of cytotoxicity

Contd.

Table 4.4 Overview of novel topical delivery system in acne (Contd.)

Novel drug delivery carrier	Drug entrapped	Method of preparation	Problem statement	Advantages
	Terbinafine hydrochloride	Solvent injection	Longer duration of treatment	Controlled release, drug targeting
Nanosuspension	Tretinoin	Precipitation	Poor water solubility and photostability	Improved drug permeation and UV irradiation stability
Nanoemulsion	Tretinoin, tetracycline	Sonication	Skin irritation, a burning sensation and peeling	Enhanced drug permeation and antibacterial activity
Nano lipid carriers	Tretinoin, tetracycline	Sonication	Skin irritation, a burning sensation, and peeling	Enhanced drug permeation and antibacterial activity
Microemulsions	Azelaic acid	—	Large and frequent dosing	Enhanced stability
	Niflumic acid	Homogenization	Weak solubility in oil and aqueous phases	Increased bioavailability at lesser concentration
	Retinoic acid	Homogenization	Systemic side effects	Enhanced skin accumulation of retinoic acid
Microspheres	Benzoyl peroxide	Emulsification	Skin irritation	Appropriate reduction in *P. acnes* count, reduced skin irritation
	Retinoid	Emulsification	Skin irritation and instability	Reduced irritation and enhanced stability
Hydrogel patches	Triclosan	Film gelation	Insufficient permeation and absorption via cutaneous route	Enhanced transdermal penetration

should be developed appending specific ligands to target the active site overcoming the biological barriers.

The encapsulation of antiacne drugs in vesicular and particulate delivery system represents an innovative alternative to minimize the related side effects, while preserving their efficacy. Novel drug delivery strategies can play a pivotal role in improving the topical delivery of antiacne agents by enhancing their dermal localization with a concomitant reduction in their side effects. Various drug delivery carriers recently explored to beat acne vulgaris are nanoparticles, liposomes, niosomes, solid lipid nanoparticles, nanoemulsions, and nanosuspensions. In fact, their ability in improving the topical delivery of antiacne agents has been very well established by *in vitro* experiments [GA Castro, 2008; AA Date, 2006]. In a recent study, solid lipid nanoparticles with chitosan containing tretinoin were prepared and characterized, which showed high encapsulation efficiency, high physical stability, and absence of cytotoxicity in keratinocytes. It also exhibited antibacterial activity against *P. acnes*, thereby increasing the therapeutic efficacy of tretinoin in the topical treatment of acne [DM Ridolfi]. Further investigations are needed, however, to allow the large scale production of novel drug delivery systems at lower costs. Finally, complementary efforts are required to validate the ability of these strategies in enhancing topical treatment of acne. A brief description of these novel carriers, their method of preparations and advantages have been summarized in Table 4.4.

REFERENCES

1. A Date, B Naik and MS Nagarsenker, "Novel drug delivery systems: potential in improving topical delivery of antiacne agents," Skin Pharmacology and Physiology, vol. 19, no. 1, pp. 2–16, 2006.

2. B Baroli, Penetration of nanoparticles and nanomaterials in the skin: fiction or reality? J. Pharm. Sci. 99 (2010) 21–50.

3. Beck RCR, Pohlmann AR, Hoffmeister C, Gallas MR, Collnot E, Schaefer UF, Guterres SS, Lehr CM. Dexamethasone-loaded nanoparticle-coated microparticles: correlation between in vitro drug release and drug transport across Caco-2 cell monolayers. Eur J Pharm Sci 2007; 67: 18–30.

4. CH Liang, TH Chou, Effect of chain length on physicochemical properties and cytotoxicity of cationic vesicles composed of phosphatidylcholines and dialkyl dimethylammonium bromides, Chem. Phys. Lipids 158 (2009) 81–90.

5. DM Ridolfi, PD Marcato, GZ Justo, L Cordi, D Machado, and N Dur´an, "Chitosan-solid lipid nanoparticles as carriers for topical delivery of

tretinoin," Colloids and Surfaces B: Biointerfaces, vol. 93, pp. 36–40, 2012.

6. FAQs: Nanotechnology, National Nanotechnology Initiative, 2010.

7. GA Castro and LAM Ferreira. "Novel vesicular and partic ulate drug delivery systems for topical treatment of acne," Expert Opinion on Drug Delivery, vol. 5, no. 6, pp. 665–679, 2008.

8. Guterres SS, Alves MP, Pohlmann AR. Polymeric nanoparticles, nanospheres and nanocapsules, for cutaneous applications. Drug Target Insights 2007; 2: 147–157.

9. J Tian, KK Wong, CM Ho, CN Lok, WY Yu, CM Che, JF Chiu, PK Tam, Topical delivery of silver nanoparticles promotes wound healing, ChemMedChem 2 (2007) 129–136.

10. M Schneider, F Stracke, S Hansen, UF Schaefer, Nanoparticles and their interactions with the dermal barrier, Dermatoendocrinology 1 (2009) 197–206.

11. Mezei M, Gulasekharam V. Liposomes: A selective drug delivery system for the topical route of administration: I: lotion dosage form. Life Sci 1980; 26: 1473–1477.

12. Osborne DW, Middleton CA, Rogers RL. Alcohol free microemulsions. J Disp Sci Technol 1988; 9: 415–423.

13. S Erdogan, Liposomal nanocarriers for tumor imaging, J. Biomed. Nanotechnol. 5 (2009) 141–150.

14. SD Roy, M Gutierrez, GL Flynn, GW Cleary, Controlled transdermal delivery of fentanyl: Characterizations of pressure-sensitive adhesives for matrix patch design, J. Pharm. Sci. 85 (1996) 491–495.

15. Schaefer H, Watts F, Brod J, Illel B. In: Scott RC, Guy RH, Hadgraft J (Eds.), Prediction of percutaneous penetration: Methods, measurements, and modelling, IBC Technical Services, London, 1990; 163–173.

III. ROLE OF SYSTEMIC THERAPY IN ACNE

INTRODUCTION

Systemic antibiotics and retinoids are the main therapeutic classes of treatment available for management of moderate to severe acne, especially if acne are unresponsive to topical treatments or have significant effect on quality of life. But in view of the rising trends of resistance antibiotic therapy is to be restricted and should not exceed 12 weeks. Also certain classes of drugs like macrolides, should be avoided as they are highly prone to resistance and have other medically important uses. Indiscriminate use in acne can lead to resistance in other indications [Leyden JJ, 2007; Sardana K 2014].

There are no differences in terms of effectivity between the different substances. So the choice has to consider resistance (rates and induction, advantage of cyclines), pharmacokinetics (advantage of second-generation cyclines), side effect profile (advantage of doxycycline and lymecycline), and costs [Falk R, 2014].

ORAL ANTIBIOTICS

Systemic antibiotics have been a mainstay in the treatment of acne, since late 1950.

- Tetracyclines and derivatives still remain the first choice.
- Macrolides.
- Co-trimoxazole and trimethoprim are other alternatives for acne [Rathi SK].

Mechanism of Action

Antibiotics target *P. acnes* and inflammation.

The anti-bacterial effect is by reducing the follicular colonization of *P. acnes*.

The anti-inflammatory effect is due to inhibition of neutrophil chemotaxis, cytokine production and macrophage function [Kubba R, 2009].

Indications

Oral antibiotics are frequently used in patients with:

1. Moderate to severe inflammatory acne
2. Acne resistant to topical treatment
3. Acne with the potential to cause pigmentary changes or permanent scarring
4. Truncal acne [Tan HH, 2003].

1. Cycline Antibiotics

Tetracyclines

Tetracycline first became available in 1953, followed by doxycycline in 1967 and minocycline in 1972, since then they became the most commonly prescribed first-line systemic antibiotic for the treatment of acne [Del Rosso JQ, 2004]. The newer generation of tetracyclines (doxycycline and minocycline) is often preferred over tetracycline, due to decreased rate of resistance and better tolerability [Leyden JJ, 2003] (Table 4.5).

MOA: Tetracyclines are antimicrobials that exert a bacteriostatic effect by interfering with protein synthesis on the 30S ribosomal subunit.

Also, they exert anti-inflammatory properties by inhibiting chemotaxis, decreasing the formation of reactive oxygen species, inhibiting proteolytic matrix metalloproteinases and downregulating pro-inflammatory cytokines [Weinberg J, 2005].

Dose

It is usually given at an initial dose of 250–500 mg once or twice per day. It is best taken on empty stomach, at least 30 min before food or 2 h afterwards, because the absorption of tetracycline is affected by food, dairy products, antacids, vitamins. Calcium or iron in food supplements combines with tetracycline, reducing their absorption.

Table 4.5 *Overview of cycline antibiotics*

Tetracyclines	Dosage	Side effects/comments
Short acting: Oxytetracycline	250–500 mg 6 hourly	To be taken on empty stomach, food and antacids decrease absorption, can cause esophagitis if swallowed dry
Intermediate acting: Demeclocycline	150–300 mg 12 hourly	High risk of photosensitivity, rarely diabetes insipidus
Long acting: Doxycycline	100 mg 12 hourly	Can be given with food and milk, safe in renal failure
Minocycline	100 mg 12 hourly	Risk of lupus, hepatitis and pneumonitis is significant

Side effects

- Gastrointestinal distress, nausea, vomiting, dyspepsia and, rarely, esophagitis and esophageal ulceration.
- Vulvovaginal candidiasis may result in 5% of the cases.
- Acneiform and fixed drug eruptions.
- Staining of growing teeth, therefore, should be avoided in pregnancy and children under the age of 9 years.
- Phototoxicity and teratogenecity.
- Rarely, Steven-Johnson syndrome can also occur [Tan HH, 2003].

Doxycycline

Doxycycline is a broad-spectrum antibiotic synthetically derived from tetracycline.

It is more lipophilic than tetracycline and has demonstrated excellent penetration into the pilosebaceous unit [Berman B, 2005].

Available as different forms:
- Doxycycline monohydrate
- Doxycycline hydrochloride hemiethanolate hemihydrates
- Doxycycline hyclate
- Doxycycline calcium

Dose

The recommended initial dose for doxycycline is 50–100 mg b.i.d.

Though not yet available in India subantimicrobial-dose doxycycline, doxycycline hyclate 20 mg may be given twice daily in acne. The conventional cycline drugs can be very effective in treating acne; however, antimicrobial level doses of these drugs can have more pronounced side effects and also contribute to the development of bacterial resistance. In order to avoid these drawbacks, doxycycline can be used for its anti-inflammatory properties through sub-antimicrobial dosing (SD) [Skidmore et al, 2003]. Patients that received SD doxycycline demonstrated significant improvement in their acne, and had no antimicrobial effect on the skin flora, as well as no increase in the number of resistant organisms. Furthermore, SD doxycycline had better tolerability and fewer side effects than antimicrobial doses of doxycycline.

Side effects

Include dental staining in <9 years, photosensitivity and teratogenic. They are similar to tetracycline but more likely to cause phototoxic reactions.

Minocycline

It is the most effective oral antibiotic in treating acne vulgaris and is considered by many to produce a more rapid and sustained clinical improvement. Minocycline being lipophilic achieves greater concentration in the tissues so is *thought* to be more effective than doxycycline, though a Cochrane review [Garner SE, 2012] did not find it superior to doxycycline.

Resistance of *P. acnes* to minocycline is considerably less than with tetracycline and doxycycline, which frequently have cross-resistance with each other [Leyden JJ, 2007]. Therefore, minocycline is more prescribed despite being expensive. *The one issue with it is the disconcerting blue- black pigmentation that often develops in some patients.*

Dose

The recommended initial dose for minocycline is 50–100 mg b.i.d followed by 50–100 mg daily. A sustained release formulation is now available in India that permits OD dosing.

Side effects

- Blue-gray skin pigmentation
- Reversible vestibular toxicity
- Drug/lupus like reactions
- Autoimmune hepatitis
- Serum sickness, vasculitis
- Dental staining in < 9 years, GI upset, teratogenic.

Oxytetracycline

It is used in a dose of 500 mg qid for 2–3 weeks, tapering to 500 mg OD and continuing according to the response.

Lymecycline

It is another member in the tetracycline family, with similar efficacy as minocycline and less side effects. Dose is 300 mg per day. It has recently been made available in India though there is no superiority in efficacy over the existing cyclines. The dose is 150 mg BD.

2. Macrolides

Macrolide antibiotics have also demonstrated efficacy in the treatment of acne.

They have a wide spectrum of activity, are well-absorbed orally, and are lipid soluble, thus penetrating well into skin structures and body fluids.

Oral macrolides, mainly erythromycin, but also roxithromycin and azithromycin, are effective in acne. However the insolicitous use of antibiotics in acne led to a large percentage of erythromycin-resistant *P. acnes* [Falk R, 2014]. This limits its use as a clear correlation between carriage of erythromycin-resistant *P. acnes* and poor clinical efficacy was demonstrated [Falk R, 2014]. Macrolides are well known to induce resistance very fast. Macrolides should therefore be only given in certain situations such as intolerance or contraindications to cyclines (e.g. pregnancy and breastfeeding). Erythromycin and clindamycin are frequently cross resistant.

MOA: They inhibit protein synthesis by binding to the 23S rRNA molecule in the 50S subunit of bacterial ribosomes.

Azithromycin

Azithromycin is a 9-methyl derivative of erythromycin that inhibits atypical intracellular pathogens such as Chlamydia and Myco-bacterium species in addition to gram-positive and gram-negative aerobic and non-aerobic bacteria including *P. acnes*.

It is characterized by rapid uptake from blood into tissues, at concentration more than 10 times of erythromycin [Kapadia N, 2004]. It also remains for prolonged period in the intracellular compartment at levels higher than the minimum inhibitory concentration for many pathogens.

It has advantages of better absorption, less drug resistance and cost effective.

Dose

It can be given in various pulse doses, 250 mg bid or 500 mg OD 3–6 days per month or 500 mg OD for 4 days every 15 days. Azithromycin, 500 mg thrice weekly for 12 weeks, is a safe and effective treatment of acne vulgaris with good patient compliance.

Efficacy

Significant improvement may be seen in 4 weeks with more than 80% reduction in the inflammatory acne lesions.

The biggest issue with this drug is that it has a high propensity to acquire resistance and as it is used for other medically important indications, like URTI, its use should be restricted to ceratin groups like children and pregnant women [Sardana K, 2014].

Side effects

- GI upset—diarrhoea, nausea, vomiting
- Drug reactions
- Antacids are known to reduce the absorption
- May interfere with the effectiveness of hormonal birth control pills.

Erythromycin

Erythromycin, commonly used for years in the treatment of acne, has been shown to be as efficacious as the tetracyclines in several studies [Gammon WR, 1996].

However, because *P. acnes* resistance to erythromycin is increasing, other macrolides and antibiotic classes are supplanting its use.

Dose

The initial dose is 250–500 mg, 2–4 times a day, reduced gradually after control is achieved.

Side effects

Include GI upset and it may increase blood levels of other drugs metabolized by the cytochrome P450 system.

Clindamycin

Dose

The dosage is 75–150 mg 1–3 times a day.

Side effects

Pseudomembranous colitis, GI upset, drug reactions.

Its use in acne is restricted and there is no rationale to use it with the known resistance to this molecule.

3. Trimethoprim/Sulfamethoxazole

In cases of treatment failure with tetracyclines and macrolide antibiotics, trimethoprim with or without sulfamethoxazole has been shown to be effective.

Its use is limited due to adverse effects. But it is successfully used as a third line agent in refractory cases of acne vulgaris.

In certain instances, patient may fail to respond to conventional antibiotics due to microbial resistance, but it has also been postulated that a high sebum excretion rate results in reduced drug concentrations in the pilosebaceous unit resulting in therapeutic failure. This is associated with many antibiotics like erythromycin, oxytetracycline, and minocycline but not trimethoprim [Layton AM, 1992]. Therefore, trimethoprim may be useful in such a situation.

Dose

Trimethoprim 300 mg BD up to 8 months.

Trimethoprim/sulfamethoxazole 480 mg once or twice daily.

Side effects

• Maculopapular rash
• Steven-Johnson syndrome

- Toxic epidermal necrolysis
- Blood dyscrasias

4. Amoxicillin

In doses from 250 mg twice daily to 500 mg three times a day, is also an alternative and may be useful during pregnancy.

ZINC SALTS IN ACNE

With the rising trends of resistance, the search is one for a viable alternate to antibiotics. Zinc fits this bill. Treatment with zinc induces a significant increase in the expression of all the markers involved in innate immunity. Inhibition of TLR2 surface expression by keratinocytes could be one of the anti-inflammatory mechanisms of zinc salts in acne. Zinc inhibits polymorphonuclear cell chemotaxis, inhibits the growth of *P. acnes*, and activates natural killer (NK) cells and the phagocytic capacity of granulocytes. Its anti-inflammatory activity in acne could also be related to a decrease in tumour necrosis factor- (TNF-α) and IL-6 production and modulation of the expression of integrins, mainly intracellular adhesion molecule-1 (ICAM-1) and leucocyte function associated antigen-3 (LFA-3) [Jarrousse V, 2007].

The therapy of acne with zinc has been found to be comparable to antibiotics including doxycyline and the dose depends on the base. A methionine based Zn has an excellent activity against acne and can be used in patients who are anxious about using antibiotic or isotretinoin. We gave a dose of methionine-based zinc complex thrice a day, though in India a tablet is available with a higher dose than can be administered twice a day [Sardana K 2010, 2014].

ANTIBIOTIC RESISTANCE

The overall incidence of *P. acne* antibiotic resistance is increasing. It is most common for tetracycline, erythromycin, clindamycin and trimethoprim.

Mechanism for antibiotic resistance: Resistance is due to point mutation at the target site in rRNA and biofilm formation {Bacteria are anchored to an internal surface of the pilosebaceous units, enveloped by an exopolysaccharide matrix, which protects them from host immune system and antibiotics.}

Antibiotic resistance should be suspected when:
- There is no clinical improvement even with good compliance
- Early response is followed by a relapse with continued treatment
- Patient has been treated with multiple courses of treatment
- If patient exhibits poor compliance [Kubba R, 2009; Sardana K].

Prevention of resistance: Combination therapy reduces chances of *P. acnes* resistance and targets more than one factor with complementary mechanism. Some simple methods can be used to avoid resistance

- Restrict the duration of antibiotics to 12 weeks.
- Avoid the use of macrolides and clindamycin.
- Antibiotics can be best used in combination with topical retinoid and benzoyl peroxide [Leyden JJ, 2003].
- BPO creams, gels and wash can be used even intermittently to help reduce the resistant strains.
- Use of systemic retinoid is another way to circumvent resistance.
- A list of combination drugs is mentioned in Table 4.6.

ISOTRETINOIN

Isotretinoin is indicated for severe cystic acne and moderate acne that are not responsive to conventional therapy or acne producing physical or psychological scarring.

It is a vitamin A analogue that inhibits sebaceous gland activity and has anti-inflammatory and anti-bacterial effects. It is naturally present in small amount in blood and tissues. It is relatively water soluble and metabolized in the liver by cytochrome P450 system.

It has high rate of permanent remission and prevention of permanent scarring in acne. It is FDA-approved for use in patients with severe, recalcitrant, nodular acne.

Table 4.6 *Combination therapy depending on type of acne*

	Moderate acne		Severe acne
	Papular/pustular	Nodulocystic	Acne conglobata/ fulminans
First line	Oral antibiotic + topical retinoid +/–BPO	Oral antibiotic + topical retinoid +/– BPO	Oral isotretinoin (may require concurrent oral steroid especially for acne fulminans)
Second line	Alternate oral antibiotic + alternate topical retinoid +/– BPO/ azelaic acid	Oral isotretinoin + alternate oral antibiotic + alternate topical retinoid +/– BPO/ azelaic acid	Dapsone + high dose oral antibiotic + topical retinoid + BPO

Mechanism of Action

- It inhibits sebum production by inhibiting sebaceous proliferation, differentiation, decreasing sebaceous gland size and down-regulation of androgen receptors in skin.
- Indirect antibacterial action due to reduction of follicular space and nutrient supply of *P. acnes*.
- Anti-inflammatory action by regulating toll-like receptors.
- Isotretinoin has been demonstrated to downregulate surface expression of TLR-2 on circulating monocytes, explaining the blunted inflammatory cytokine response to *P. acnes* [Dispenza MC, 2012].

Efficacy of Isotretinoin

About 60–85% of patients are expected to achieve a clinical cure rate after 20 weeks of treatment [Lehmann HP, 2001]. In most patients, isotretinoin yields skin improvement by *third* month of treatment [Manolache L, 2005]. Certain group of patients may require second isotretinoin course or oral antibiotics after the isotretinoin treatment.

Patient Selection

It is very important to determine whether he/she is an appropriate isotretinoin candidate:

- All womens of child bearing age should be counselled regarding the adverse effects of isotretinoin on fetus.
- The patient medical history must be evaluated.
- Patients with known hypersensitivity to isotretinon or any of its components should not be treated with isotretinoin.
- History of alcohol intake should be evaluated.
- History of patients, to rule any psychiatric disorder or suicidal ideation.
- History of pre-existing medical conditions should be taken.

Dose

Isotretinoin is lipophilic molecule which is optimally absorbed when taken with a fatty meal.

The generally recommended dose is 0.5–1 mg/kg/day in one or two daily doses to reach a target cumulative dose of 120 mg/kg. Therapy is typically initiated at 0.5 mg/kg/day to avoid initial flare and then increased as tolerated to 1mg/kg/day to limit side effects that are generally dose related. When prescribed this way, treatment course lasts for 20 weeks. Alternatively, low-dose isotretinoin can be used for longer periods with a cumulative dose of 120–150 mg/kg over the treatment course [Arshdeep, 2013].

Low Dose Isotretinoin

This form of therapy should be restricted to moderate grades of acne as in severe cases there is a high degree of relapse rate. The dose is 0.3–0.5 mg/kg and can be given daily, alternate day or as an intermittent therapy and has markedly less side-effects [Sardana K, 2010]. In some cases of adult acne a low-dose isotretinoin for 1–2 days of each week is an useful method of keeping the disease under control.

Intermittent or variable dose: Intermittent dosed isotretinoin at 0.5 mg/kg per day for 1 week out of every 4 weeks for 6 months can be given for adult acne.

High dose: Since many isotretinoin side effects are dose dependent, use of high dose isotretinoin is very challenging. High dose isotretinoin 1 mg/kg/day has been explored and has a very low recurrence rate than those treated with 0.5 mg/kg/day [Cunliffe WJ, 1997].

Relapse

Isotretinoin can approach a cure in approximately 40% of treated patients while the majority achieve improvestment [White GM, 1998].

Relapse may occur, especially in younger patients, males and those with truncal acne. However, they can often be managed with oral antibiotics and topical agents. If acne remains severe, a repeat course of isotretinoin may be considered [Azoulay L, 2007].

Patients who do not reach the cumulative target dose. Or discontinue therapy prematurely, are more likely to relapse.

Adverse Effects

Adverse effects associated with isotretinoin are dose dependent and are reversible.

- Cheilitis and mucocutaneous dryness are most common.
- Dyslipidemia, increase transaminase levels, pancytopenia, nausea, diarrhoea, idiopathic intracranial hypertension, arthralgia and myalgia.
- It is teratogenic and contraindicated during pregnancy. Birth defects, abnormal neurological functioning, retinoid embryopathy are known to occur.
- Inflammatory bowel disease.
- Psychological effects include depression, psychosis, suicidal ideation.
- Tetracyclines should be avoided in combination with isotretinoin due to possible risk of benign intracranial hypertension.
- Skeletal abnormalities including DISH (diffuse idiopathic skeletal hyperostosis), calcification of ligaments, osteoporosis and premature fusion of epiphysis.

- Hepatotoxicity and hepatitis.
- Rarely, glomerulonephritis due to drug hypersensitivity.

Contraindications

Absolute
- Pregnancy and lactation

Relative
- Hyperlipidaemia
- Children
- Diabetes mellitus
- Liver disease
- Raised intracranial pressure
- Suicidal ideation

Acute Flare of Acne, Early in a Course and Its Management

- An acute flare in the course of isotretinoin is a recognized problem. Therefore, a physician should inform this patient accordingly and provide a fast track follow up.
- Predisposing risk factors for the flare include: The presence of macro-comedones and severe acne with nodules, male gender.
- *Prevention*: It is recommended that patients are started on a lower dose of isotretinoin and then escalated as tolerated.

  Oral corticosteroids (e.g. prednisone dosed at 0.5 mg/kg/day for 2–6 weeks) may be administered at the same time as initiating isotretinoin to prevent this flare [Chivot M, 2001; Demircay Z, 2008]. Another option is to initiate at a lower dose (0.5 mg/kg/day) or administer concomitant NSAID.

  Management: Macrocomedones should be identified before systemic isotretinoin is started.

  An antibiotic can be used in combination with isotretinoin such as erythromycin 1 g daily or trimethoprim 200–300 mg BD.

  If acne is very inflammatory, then steroids may be required [e.g. 0.5–1 mg/kg/day for 2–3 weeks] [Alison L, 2009]. In other patients it may be appropriate to increase the dose of isotretinoin provided that the side effects are tolerated.

CONCLUSION

Among *antibiotics*, tetracyclines have been the mainstay for first-line oral therapy in acne, but it is important to be aware of other potential options that are available in this group, e.g. sub-antimicrobial dose doxycycline. Minocycline and trimethoprim-sulphamethoxazole remains good option for second line treatment in cases of refractory acne.

Within the macrolide class, azithromycin appears to be a viable option, *in children and pregnant female.*

Isotretinoin is highly effective, well-tolerated acne treatment that has revolutionized the treatment for severe nodulocystic acne.

Novel agents like zinc can be used as they have a proven efficacy in pustular acne and also do not cause resistance.

REFERENCES

1. Alison L. The use of isotretinoin in acne. Dermatoendocrinol 2009; 162–169.
2. Amnesteem (Isotretinoin Capsules USP) [pakage insert]. Morgantown, WV: Mylan Pharmaceuticals, Inc. 2010.
3. Arshdeep, De D. What's new in the management of acne? Indian J Dermatol Venereol Leprol 2013;79:279–87.
4. Azoulay L, Oraichi D, Berard A. Isotretinoin therapy and the incidence of acne relapse: a nested case-control study. Br J Dermatol. 2007; 157(6):1240–8.
5. Berman B, Zell D. Subantimicrobial dose doxycycline: a unique treatment for rosacea. Cutis. 2005; 75:19–24.
6. Chivot M. Acne flare-up and deterioration with oral isotretinoin. Ann Dermatol Venereol 2001; 128:224–228.
7. Cunliffe WJ, van de Kerkhof PCM, Caputo R, et al. Roaccutane treatment guidelines: result of an international survey. Dermatology 1997; 194:351–357.
8. Del Rosso JQ. A status report on the use of sub-antimicrobial dose doxycycline: a review of the biologic and antimicrobial effects of the tetracyclines. Cutis. 2004; 74:118–122.
9. Demircay Z, Kus S, Sur H. Predictive factors for acne flare during isotretinoin treatment. Eur J Dermatol 2008; 18(40):452–456.
10. Dispenza MC, Wolpert EB, Cilliland KL, et al. Systemic isotretinoin therapy normalizes exaggerated TLR-2-mediated innate immune responses in acne patients. J Invest Dermtol 2012; 132:2198–2205.
11. Falk R. Ochsendorf . Oral Antibiotics . C.C. Zouboulis et al. (eds.), Pathogenesis and Treatment of Acne and Rosacea,DOI 10.1007/978-3-540-69375-8_60, © Springer-Verlag Berlin Heidelberg 2014.
12. Gammon WR, Meyer C, Lantis S, et al. Comparative study of oral erythromycin versus oral tetracycline in the treatment of acne vulgaris: a double-blind study. J Am Acad Dermatol. 1986; 14:183–186.
13. Garner SE, Eady A, Bennett C, Newton JN, Thomas K, Popescu CM. Minocycline for acne vulgaris: efficacy and safety. Cochrane Database Syst Rev. 2012 Aug 15; 8:CD002086.
14. Jarrousse V, Castex-Rizzi N, Khammari A, Charveron M, Dréno B. Zinc salts inhibit in vitro Toll-like receptor 2 surface expression by keratinocytes. European Journal of Dermatology, 2007; 17(6):492–496.

15. Kapadia N, Talib A. Acne treated successfully with azithromycin. Int J Dermatol. 2004; 43:766–767.
16. Kubba R, Bajaj A K, Thappa D M, Sharma R, Vedamurthy M, Dhar S. Antibiotic resistance in acne. Indian J Dermatol Venereol Leprol 2009; 75, Suppl S1:37–38.
17. Kubba R, Bajaj A K, Thappa D M, Sharma R, Vedamurthy M, Dhar S. Oral antibiotics. Indian J Dermatol Venereol Leprol 2009; 75, Suppl S1:35–6.
18. Layton AM, Hughes BR, Macdonald-Hull S, et al. Seborrhoea-an indicator of poor clinical response in acne patients treated with antibiotics. Clin Ex Dermatol. 1992; 17:173–175.
19. Lehmann HP, Andrews JS, Robinson KA, Holloway VL, Goodman SN. Management of acne. US Agency for Healthcare Research and Quality (AHRQ) Evidence report/Technology Assessment Number 17; Sept 2001.
20. Leyden JJ, Del Rosso JQ, Webster GF. Clinical considerations in the treatment of acne vulgaris and other inflammatory skin disorders: focus on antibiotic resistance. Cutis. 2007; 79:9–25.
21. Leyden JJ. A review of the use of combination therapies for the treatment of acne vulgaris. J Am Acad Dermatol. 2003; 49(3):S200–10.
22. Manolache L, Benea V, Dumitrescu R, Diaconu J. Acne treatment with low-doses of systemic isotretinoin. Dermatol Klin 2005; 7(1): 7–10.
23. Rathi SK. Acne vulgaris treatment : The Current Scenario. Indian J Dermatol 2011; 56:7–13
24. Sardana K, Chugh S, Garg VK. The role of zinc in acne and prevention of resistance: have we missed the "base" effect? Int J Dermatol. 2014 Jan; 53(1):125–7.
25. Sardana K, Garg VK. An observational study of methionine-bound zinc with antioxidants for mild to moderate acne vulgaris. Dermatol Ther. 2010 Jul-Aug; 23(4):411–8.
26. Sardana K, Garg VK. Antibiotic resistance in acne: is it time to look beyond antibiotics and Propionobacterium acnes? Int J Dermatol. 2014 Jul; 53(7):917–9.
27. Sardana K, Garg VK. Efficacy of low-dose isotretinoin in acne vulgaris. Indian J Dermatol Venereol Leprol 2010; 76:7–13.
28. Skidmore R, Kovach R, Walker C, et al. Effects of sub-antimicrobial doxycycline in the treatment of moderate acne. Arch Dermatol. 2003; 139:459–64.
29. Tan HH. Antibacterial therapy for acne. Am J Dermatol. 2003; 4:307–314.
30. Weinberg J. The anti-inflammatory effects of tetracyclines. Cutis. 2005; 75:6–11.
31. White GM, Chen W, Yao J, Wolde-Tsadik G. Recurrence rates after the first course of isotretinoin. Arch Dermatol. 1998; 134:376–8.

IV. HORMONAL TREATMENT IN ACNE

INTRODUCTION

Androgens play an important role in acne vulgaris [Zouboulis CC, 1993], though not all studies have been able to demonstrate them biochemically in persistent. This is as 3-α-androstanediol glucuronide is the true indicator of peripheral androgenic abnormality, which is relevant in acne, hisrustism and FPHL. Most studies published in dermatology journals do not look at this hormone.

A study [Vexiau P, 2000] found that the severity of female-pattern androgenetic alopecia is closely related to observed levels of two of parameters (3 alpha-diol G and SHBG). This has also been noted both in females with hirsutism [Carmina E and Lobo RA, 2001] and males [Lookingbill DP, 1998] with chest hair density and acne. Patients with acne and those with isolated hirsutism showed significantly decreased sex hormone binding globulin plasma levels. However, while all patients with hirsutism showed increased plasma values of 3 alpha-androstanediol and its glucuronide, all patients with acne showed plasma levels within the normal range, independently of the precursor plasma levels. Thus it was proposed that dihydrotestosterone is further reduced to 3 alpha-androstanediol and its glucuronide only in hirsute patients but not in acne patients. These results suggest that dihydrotestosterone may undergo different metabolic pathways at skin levels and support the hypothesis that the two clinical manifestations may be the expression of the different metabolic fate of dihydrotestosterone itself. Thus 3 alpha-androstanediol and its glucuronide cannot be always be used as plasma markers of target-tissue produced androgens in all hyperandrogenic conditions [Toscano V, 1993].

Hormonal treatments are effective in acne by lowering circulating and local androgen levels and opposing their effects on the sebaceous gland and probably on the follicular keratinocytes as well. Hormonal treatments, should be directed at the cause, thus if the source is the ovaries, OCP are ideal, while if it is the adrenal gland, steroids are needed. In case no defect is found as is the case in most patients spironolactone which is an androgen receptor blocker is a useful modality (Table 4.7).

INDICATIONS OF HORMONAL THERAPY

Hormonal therapy may be useful for acne in selected cases [Gollnick H, 2003]. It is important to note that hormonal therapy can be very effective in females with acne whether their serum androgens are *abnormal or not* [Thiboutot D, 2004]. This is as the problem in most

Table 4.7 Indications of hormonal treatment	
Females	*Males*
• When oral contraception is desirable may be used in cases of proven	Low-dose oral glucocorticoids adrenal hyperandrogenism
• As an alternative when repeated courses of isotretinoin are needed (persistent acne)	
• Women whose acne is not responding to conventional therapy	
• Polycystic ovary syndrome	
• When there are clinical signs of hyperandrogenism, such as androgenic alopecia and seborrhea, acne, hirsutism, alopecia (SAHA) syndrome	
• Late-onset acne (acne tarda)	
• Proven ovarian hyperandrogenism	
• Proven adrenal hyperandrogenism	

cases may be at the end organ level and receptor blocking drugs are immensely useful in such cases.

In males (Table 4.7) the only indication is CAH (congenital adrenal hyperplasia) and is treated by low-dose glucocorticoids. NCCAH is a cause of persistent acne in females, is not common. In a study from Greece of the 146 women studied only 6 had NCCAH (Trakakis E et al, 2013). There was no statistical significant difference in the frequency of peripubertal acne between NCCAH group of patients (6.4%) and patients with hyperandrogenemia of other aetiology (93%), mainly ovarian. However, there was a statistical significant difference in the prevalence of acne at the time of clinical examination between the two groups (P = 0.04). Acne was present in 83.3% of women with NCCAH vs. 41.02% of women in the hyperandrogenic group without NCCAH. Nervertheless, NCCAH is not a very common cause of persistent acne in clinical practice.

Polycystic ovary syndrome (PCOS) may possibly be the most common cause of hormonal acne in females, with an underlying biochemical evidence of hyperandrogenism. An oral contraceptive pill therapy is the first line of therapy for hirsutism and acne in women with PCOS. Drospirenone/EE- and CPA/EE-containing oral contraceptives are effective in PCOS-associated acne therapy [Frangos J, 2008].

DRUGS

Anti-androgens or androgen receptor blockers are defined as agents that inhibit directly the binding of dihydrotestosterone (DHT) to its receptor in a competitive way. They include cyproterone acetate, drospirenone, and spironolactone (Table 4.8).

Cyproterone Acetate

Cyproterone acetate (CPA) is the only anti-androgen that also has an anti-gonadotropin action by inhibiting ovulation.

1. It inhibits the production of follicle-stimulating hormone (FSH) and luteinizing hormone (LH)
2. It inhibits the ovarian function
3. The serum androgen levels are reduced
4. It inhibits the binding of 5α-dihydrotestosterone (DHT) to the androgen receptor and it reduces the activity of 5α-reductase that catalyzes the transformation of testosterone to DHT. CPA (10, 50 mg) treatment has been used in acne.

Regimen

CPA should begin on the first day of the menstrual period. It may be given alone (at a dose of 50–100 mg daily) or in combination with ethinyl estradiol (EE) in the form of an oral contraceptive (CPA 2 mg/ EE 35 µg). CPA (even at low doses of 12.5 mg, that is, ¼ of the 50 mg tablet) may be added to the fixed combination of CPA 2 mg/EE 35 µg during the first 10 or 15 days of the menstrual cycle, in order to avoid menstrual irregularities caused during treatment with

Table 4.8 *Overview of hormonal treatment in acne tarda*		
Ovarian cause	Estrogens/OCP	1. Suppression of the ovarian production of androgens by suppressing gonadotropin release
		2. Stimulation of hepatic synthesis of sex hormone-binding globulin (SHBG)
	GnRH agonists	Inhibition of ovarian androgen production
Adrenal	Oral glucocortico-steroids	Blocking of adrenal androgen production
End organ	Anti-androgens	1. Inhibition of ovulation
		2. Blocking androgen receptors
		3. Inhibition of 5α-reductase

CPA alone. CPA/EE-containing oral contraceptives and CPA are not approved for use in the USA but are approved in Europe and India.

Side effects

The most frequent side effect is amenorrhea or oligomenorrhea. Other side effects include nausea, vomiting, fluid retention, leg edema, headache, and melasma. CPA has also been associated with tiredness, headache, liver dysfunction, shortness of breath, and blood clotting disorders.

Spironolactone

Spironolactone may be used for female patients with therapy-resistant acne, although it has not been approved for this disorder. It has been used in doses ranging from 25 to 100 mg daily [Akamatsu H]. Most commonly, spironolactone is used in countries where no other anti-androgens are available.

Use

In general, it should be reserved for cases resistant to conventional therapy. Spironolactone may be combined with an oral contraceptive. It functions both as an androgen receptor blocker and an inhibitor of 5 α-reductase. Response in acne may take as long as 3 months as with other hormonal therapies.

Side effects

Adverse effects are dose dependent. Low doses such as 25–50 mg daily are generally well tolerated. It may be associated with hyperkalemia, menstrual irregularity, breast tenderness, headache, and fatigue. A recent study found that the risk of hyperkalemia is low (0.72%). It is contraindicated in women at increased risk of breast cancer. Treatment with spironolactone during pregnancy may lead to abnormalities of the male fetal genitalia, such as hypospadias.

Oral Contraceptives

Oral contraceptives (OC) contain an estrogen (EE) and a progestin. Progestins are used in order to avoid the risk of endometrial cancer associated with unopposed estrogens. The progestins contained in OC include estranes and gonanes, which are derivatives of 19-nortestosterone, CPA, and a novel progestin, drospirenone.

MOA

Drospirenone, a progestin derived from 17 α-spironolactone, has anti-androgenic as well as anti-mineralocorticoid activity [Thorneycroft I, 2002]. EE may have anti-androgenic effects either by suppressing the secretion of pituitary gonadotropins, thereby inhibiting production of ovarian androgens, or by increasing liver synthesis of sex hormone-binding globulin (SHBG), which reduces the circulating free testosterone level [Lucky AW, 1997].

Use

In Europe, the OC containing CPA 2 mg/EE 35 mg is approved for the treatment of acne. In the USA, there are three FDA-approved OC for acne therapy, namely the combinations of norgestimate/EE, norethindrone/EE, and 3 mg drospirenone/20 mg EE.

OC are approved for acne treatment in female patients older than 14 years old, and guidelines suggest that OC treatment is discontinued 3–4 cycles *after* acne improvement [Junkins-Hopkins JM, 2010]. In India, all the three OCP are available, though I prefer the 3 mg drospirenone/20 µg EE preparation. A study with drospirenone 3 mg/EE 30 µg showed a higher efficacy in total acne lesion reduction compared to norgestimate/EE 35 µg and a similar efficacy to CPA 2 mg/EE 35 µg [Thomeycroft H, 2004]. A randomized, placebo-controlled study of drospirenone 3 mg/EE 20 µg for 6 months in 538 women (14–35 years old) with moderate acne showed efficacy in both inflammatory acne lesions and comedones [Maloney JM, 2009].

Importantly, OCP are *not* to be used as monotherapy, thus when they are combined with existing agents, and then the results achieved in hormonal acne are faster and more satisfactory. I frequently combine OCP with low dose isotretinoin, with excellent results. The OCP obviates the risk of unwanted pregnancy that is a concern with isotretinoin.

Side effects

Oral contraceptives are contraindicated in women with a history of clotting disorder, thrombophlebitis, cerebrovascular disease, coronary occlusion, abnormal vaginal bleeding, impaired liver function, migraine, in smokers over age 35, and in individuals at increased risk of breast cancer.

The most serious side effect of oral contraceptives, thrombo-embolism, has largely been eliminated by the reduced doses of estrogen used in modern formulations. The incidence of other serious adverse effects, such as hypertension that follow the use of estrogens, is rare in young healthy females. Frequently reported adverse effects include metrorrhagia, nausea, vomiting, breast tenderness, headache, edema of the venous system of the lower extremities, and weight gain. These are often transient and resolve after the first few months of therapy.

In case of combination therapy with oral antibiotics and oral contra-ceptives, there is no scientific evidence supporting the effect of antibiotics to reduce either blood levels and/or the effectiveness of oral contraceptives, with the exception of rifampin (rifampicin)-like drugs.

Oral Glucocorticosteroids

The symptomatology of NCCAH is important in cases of acne. Moran et al, 2000 reviewing the distribution of symptoms in 220 women from 11 centers found that, hirsutism after the age of 10 years was present in 59% and acne in 33% of women. Male pattern baldness in females has been reported to be the sole symptomatic sign of NCCAH. Refractory acne can have underlying NCCAH (Degitz K, 2003) and respond to glucocorticoid therapy. In one small study, treatment with dexamethasone 0.25 mg orally every evening reversed acne in 3 months but hirsutism required up to 30 months of treatment for resolution [New M, 1996].

Low-dose oral glucocorticosteroids may be useful in therapy of acne in patients with well-documented adrenal hyperandrogenism. Low-dose glucocorticoids are most commonly used to treat male or female patients with classic or late-onset congenital adrenal hyperplasia.

Low-dose prednisolone (2.5–5 mg/day) or low-dose dexamethasone (0.25–0.75 mg) can be given orally at bedtime), although the latter incurs a higher risk of adrenal suppression. The DHEAS level is used to monitor therapy and a target is a level of approximately 70 µg per dL, at which time the drug should be stopped.

Gonadotropin-Releasing Hormone (GnRH Agonists)

These include buserelin, nafarelin, or leuprolide, and they block androgen production in the ovary.

They block ovulation by interrupting the cyclic release of FSH and LH from the pituitary. They are available in injectable and nasal spray forms and have proven to be efficacious in treating acne and hirsutism, but drawbacks that limit their use include the high cost and side effects like osteoporosis.

Finasteride

5α-reductase inhibitors can be classified as type 1, type 2, and type 1/2 dual inhibitors, depending on which isoenzyme of 5α-reductase they inhibit. 5α-reductase (5α-R) is the enzyme that catalyzes the conversion of testosterone to DHT. Type 1 5α-reductase exists predominantly in the skin, where its activity is concentrated in the sebaceous glands and is significantly higher in sebaceous glands from the face and scalp compared with nonacne-prone areas. Type 25α-reductase exists predominantly in the prostate and within hair follicles.

Thus, finasteride, does not have a marked effect on the type 1 receptors, which is a reason that it is not effective in hormonal acne. A recent study though found finasteride 5 mg to be effective in 9/12 women with normal serum levels of free testosterone suffering from acne or alopecia [*Kohler C*].

CONCLUSION

It has been the experience of most authors who have worked in the field of hormonal acne that, it is a common cause of persistent and refractory acne in women. Identification of a definite hormonal defect is not always possible in all cases, but the fact that such patients respond to anti-androgens and receptor blockers is the proof that there is a central or peripheral androgenic defect. PCOS is the most common cause of androgen-induced acne, and apart from treating acne, with OCP, nutrition and lifestyle changes may be effective. It is also important to recognize that hormonal therapy, when added to an acne regimen, cannot only improve the patient's acne but in many cases can also obviate the need for chronic antibiotic therapy or repeat courses of isotretinoin.

REFERENCES

1. Akamatsu H, Zouboulis CC, Orfanos CE. Spironolactone directly inhibits proliferation of cultured human facial sebocytes and acts antagonistically to testosterone and 5-alpha-dihydrotestosterone in vitro. J Invest Dermatol. 1993; 100:660–2.
2. Carmina E and Lobo RA. Hirsutism, alopecia and acne. In Becker KL (ed.) Principles and Practice of Endocrinology and Metabolism, 3rd edn. Philadelphia, PA: Lippincott Williams and Wilkins, 2001;991–995.
3. Degitz K, Placzek M, Arnold B, et al. Congenital adrenal hyperplasia and acne in male patients. Br J Dermatol. 2003; 148:1263–1266.
4. Frangos J, Alavian CN, Kimball AB. Acne and oral contraceptives: update on women's health screening guidelines. J Am Acad Dermatol. 2008; 58:781–6.
5. Gollnick H, Cunliffe W, Berson D, et al. Management of acne. J Am Acad Dermatol. 2003; 49:S20–5.
6. Junkins-Hopkins JM. Hormone therapy for acne. J Am Acad Dermatol. 2010; 62:486–8.
7. Lookingbill DP, Egan N, Santen RJ, Demers LM. Correlation of serum 3 alpha-androstanediol glucuronide with acne and chest hair density in men. J Clin Endocrinol Metab. 1988 Nov; 67(5):986–91.
8. Lucky AW, Henderson TA, Olson WH, et al. Effectiveness of norgestimate and ethinyl estradiol in treating moderate acne vulgaris. J Am Acad Dermatol. 1997; 37:746–54.

9. Maloney JM, Dietze Jr P, Watson D, et al. A randomized controlled trial of a low-dose combined oral contraceptive containing 3 mg drospirenone plus 20 microg ethinylestradiol in the treatment of acne vugaris: lesion counts, investigator ratings and subject self-assessment. J Drugs Dermatol. 2009; 8:837–44.

10. Moran C, Azziz R, Carmina E, et al. 21-hydroxylase-deficient nonclassic adrenal hyperplasia is a progressive disorder: a multicenter study. Am J Obstet Gynecol. 2000; 183:1468–74.

11. New M. Infertility and androgen excess in nonclassical 21-hydroxylase deficiency. Symposium on the Ovary: Regulation, Dysfunction and Treatment; Marco Island. Jan 25-27, 1996; pp. 195–198.

12. Thorneycroft I. Evolution of progestins. Focus on the novel progestin drospirenone. J Reprod Med. 2002; 47 Suppl 11:975–80.

13. Thomeycroft H, Gollnick H, Schellschmidt I. Superiority of a combined contraceptive containing drospirenone to a triphasic preparation containing norgestimate in acne treatment. Cutis. 2004; 74:123–30.

14. Vogt C, Dericks-Tan JS, Kuhl H, Taubert HD. Is 3 alpha, 17 beta-androstanediol-glucuronide a diagnostic marker in women with androgenic manifestations? Gynecol Endocrinol. 1992 Jun; 6(2): 85–90.

15. Thiboutot D. Acne: hormonal concepts. Clin Dermatol. 2004; 22:419–28.

16. Toscano V, Balducci R, Bianchi P, Guglielmi R, Mangiantini A, Rossi FG,Colonna LM, Sciarra F. Two different pathogenetic mechanisms may play a role in acne and in hirsutism. Clin Endocrinol (Oxf). 1993 Nov; 39(5):551–6.

17. Trakakis E, Papadavid E, Dalamaga M, Koumaki D, Stavrianeas N, Rigopoulos D,Creatsas G, Kassanos D. Prevalence of non classical congenital adrenal hyperplasia due to 21-hydroxylase deficiency in Greek women with acne: a hospital-based cross-sectional study. J Eur Acad Dermatol Venereol. 2013 Nov; 27(11):1448–51.

18. Vexiau P, Chaspoux C, Boudou P, Fiet J, Abramovici Y, Rueda MJ, Hardy N, Reygagne P. Role of androgens in female-pattern androgenetic alopecia, either alone or associated with other symptoms of hyperandrogenism. Arch Dermatol Res. 2000 Dec; 292(12):598–604.

V. CLEANSERS, SUNSCREENS AND COSMETICS IN ACNE

INTRODUCTION

Acne patients are a highly motivated patient class, who are obviously concerned about their body image. The face being the "passport to society" is the object of attention and apart from the medications given by dermatologists various other cosmetics are invariably used, to mask, clean or conceal the acne lesions. We will examine the common agents used and their impact on acne.

SUNSCREENS AND ACNE

Many patients note the occurrence of 'breakouts' following the use of sunscreens. These patients typically present with perifollicular papules and pustules in a random distribution over the face. This eruption appears within 24–48 hours after wearing a facial sunscreen.

Most of the sunscreens on the market today are based primarily on UVB-absorbing ingredients, such as octyl methoxycinnamate, oxybenzone, homosalate, etc. Many also have UVA-absorbing ingredients, such as avobenzone, titanium dioxide, or zinc oxide, as secondary sunscreens. All of the UVB sunscreens and avobenzone function by transforming ultraviolet radiation to heat energy through a process known as resonance delocalization. This heat energy is appreciated by many patients who will state that they do not like wearing sunscreens, since the gels or lotions make them feel hot. In some patients, I believe that the increased sweating induced by the sunscreens accompanied by the warm sunny humid weather cause increased activity by the eccrine glands. This may cause miliaria rubra that may be magnified by the occlusive nature of the water-resistant, rubproof product that some sunscreens claim to be nowadays.

We have shown that acne actually worsens in summer with the concomitant increased humidity, thus most of the sunscreen, bases, which are lotion, creams, hydrogels, with various occlusive properties, can actually cause acne (cosmetic). Though sunscreen use does not prevent or modify the course of acne, it is a common adjunct. This is as retinoids increase the photoerythema and Indian skin is predisposed to PIH. Thus apart from avoiding sun exposure, a mat based sunscreen is ideal in such cases. In India though, the patients who cannot afford to buy sunscreens are usually indoors, while those who cant afford them are usually in jobs that expose them to the sun. With our intrinsic pigmented skin, sunscreen use is more of a "media" drive craze than a necessity and I do not routinely advise them in all acne patients.

ACNE CLEANSERS

Acne cleansers utilize the same surfactants found in cleansing products for the general population, but in addition focus on reducing the oiliness of the face. Commonly used agents like, soaps, are some of the major cleansers used, though they have an alkaline pH of 9–10. Many of the milder acne soaps are composed of synthetic detergents, known as syndets. These cleansers contain less than 10% soap with a more neutral pH adjusted to 5.5–7.0. But in acne, most popular soaps are alkaline and have triclosan, a potent antibacterial helpful in acne that is considered an acne treatment in Europe, but is not listed in the Acne Monograph in the USA. A very popular anti-acne foaming facewash contains cocamidopropyl betainamide MEA chloride which is a milder and environment friendly surfactant than SLS.

Facial scrubs contain the cleansing ingredients previously discussed, but may add physical scrubbing granules designed to aid in removal of comedonal plugs composed of polyethylene beads, aluminium oxide, ground fruit pits, or sodium tetraborate decahydrate granules [Mills OH, 1979]. Polyethylene beads are popular as they have smooth spheres that do not damage the skin surface. Other useful agents are sodium tetraborate decahydrate granules, which dissolve during the scrubbing process when mixed with water limiting the length of time the granules can produce exfoliation.

The active surfactants that are effective at removing the sebum, bacteria, and environmental dirt, are invariably supplemented by a variety of acne treatment ingredients that may be added as active ingredients in the formulation. These ingredients include benzoyl peroxide, salicylic acid, sulphur, and hydroxy acids.

1. Benzoyl Peroxide

Benzoyl peroxide is an organic peroxide consisting of two benzoyl groups joined by a peroxide group prepared by reacting sodium peroxide with benzoyl chloride to yield benzoyl peroxide and sodium chloride. Benzoyl peroxide has many properties pertinent to acne, including antibacterial, anti-inflammatory, and comedolytic effects. Bojar RA had shown that the use of 5% benzoyl peroxide can effect a 2-log 10 decrease in *P. acnes* concentration after 2 days. This type of bacterial killing may *not* be seen with benzoyl peroxide cleansers that have a *short skin contact time;* however, benzoyl peroxide cleansers can suppress the development of resistant organisms [Leyden JJ, 2007]. It must be emphasised that there is a method that has to be adopted to help in decrease in *P. acnes* counts. Leyden had demonstrated a decrease in the counts of resistant *P. acnes* strains over 12 weeks with the BPO 6% cleanser if the prescribed method is followed.

Thus the subjects wet their faces and liberally applied the cleanser while working up a *full lather* with *particular attention given to the forehead region*. They gently massaged the cleanser into the skin for 10 to 20 seconds, then rinsed their faces with water and patted dry. Recently a BP 9.8% emollient foam in reducing *P. acnes* levels on the back with 2 minutes of skin contact time and had comparative results with a BP 5.3% "leave-on" emollient foam formulation. Short contact therapy utilizing a 2-minute skin contact time with BP 9.8% emollient foam used once daily over a 2-week duration was highly effective in reducing the quantity of *P. acnes* organisms on the back and provided comparable colony count reduction to "leave on" therapy using BP 5.3% emollient foam [Leyden, 2102]. Thus for larger and difficult to reach areas like the back this may be a viable option.

2. Salicylic Acid

The other major comedolytic used as an active in OTC cleansers is salicylic acid in concentrations up to 2%, as allowed by the United States Acne Monograph [Eady EA, 1996]. Salicylic acid is a colorless crystalline oil soluble phenolic compound originally derived from the willow tree Salix. It is a beta hydroxy acid where the OH group is adjacent to the carboxyl group. Salicylic acid can penetrate into the follicle and dislodge the comedonal plug from the follicular lining. It does *not* kill *P. acnes*, however, and does not prevent the development of antibiotic resistance. The effects of salicylic acid in a cleanser formulation are less than a leave-on formulation due to the reduction in contact time. Some salicylic acid formulations try to overcome this brief contact by using smaller particle size and depositing the material into the pores during facial rinsing [Chen T, 2006].

3. Sulphur

The oldest treatment for acne predating benzoyl peroxide and salicylic acid is sulphur, which is *bacteriostatic* [Gupta AK, 2004]. It is a yellow, non-metallic element that has been used in OTC acne preparations. The mechanism of action for sulphur is not totally understood, but it is thought to interact with cysteine in the stratum corneum causing a reduction in sulphur to hydrogen sulphide. Hydrogen sulphide in turn degrades keratin producing the keratolytic effect of sulphur [Lin AN]. Sulphur has been labeled as a comedogen, but this is controversial. It is available in concentrations of 3–8 % in OTC acne formulations, but has a characteristic foul odor and yellow color. Decolorized, deodorized sulphur is available, but it is not commonly used in acne cleansers.

4. Hydroxy Acids

Hydroxy acids, such as glycolic acid, have also been used in acne treatments as desquamating agents. Glycolic acid is the smallest alpha hydroxy acid appearing as a colorless, odourless, hygroscopic crystalline solid. While glycolic acid can be obtained from the fermentation of sugarcane, it is more commonly synthesized by reacting chloroacetic acid with sodium hydroxide followed by re-acidication. No acne claims can be made regarding hydroxy acids in the USA because glycolic acid is not listed on the acne monograph. The efficacy of glycolic acid in treating acne is related to the free acid concentration. The free acid is able to dissolve the ionic bonds between the corneocytes forming the stratum corneum. This desquamation can remove the comedonal plugs; however, the water-soluble glycolic acid cannot enter the oily milieu of the pore.

Thus its my opinion as is the opinion of a leading authority on cosmetics in acne, Dr ZD Draelos, that in acne saliylic acid is superior to GA. Thus if such a wash is to prescribed, a SA based wash is ideal.

ACNE MOISTURISERS

Topical therapies, including SA, BP, retinoids, and antibiotics are effective in managing acne, but are associated with local adverse effects, such as irritation and dryness. A concomitant use of moisturizers can enhance efficacy, alleviate dryness, and improve skin comfort. The study by Laquieze et al, (2006) showed that using moisturizers provided a significant improvement in skin dryness and comfort to the patients who were treated with oral or topical isotretinoin. Most acne moisturisers contain SA. However, SA is likely to cause local skin peeling when used at concentrations of 2% or more. Similarly, BP and retinols are regarded as irritative agents. BP has greater activity than topical (iso) tretinoin against inflammatory lesions while retinoids work well for comedolytic effects and decrease sebum excretion. It has been shown that the adjunctive use of a moisturizer (Cetaphil®, Galderma Laboratories, LP) improved local tolerance of adapalene gel.

Dimethicone and *glycerin* are the most common ingredients found in acne moisturisers. Dimethicone and cyclomethicone are silicone derivatives and usually used in oil-free facial moisturizers [Del Rosso JQ, 2009]. The term "oil-free" implies that this substance does not contain either mineral oil or vegetable oil. Dimethicone reduces TEWL without a greasy feel and contains both occlusive and emollient properties. It is suitable for acne and sensitive patients as it is noncomedogenic and hypoallergenic. Cyclomethicone is a thicker silicone that has similar properties as dimethicone. Other ingredients like petrolatum, lanolin, and mineral oil, which have a sticky feel. *Glycerin* is the most effective humectant available to increase stratum corneum hydration. If the concentration of glycerin is too high, it will create a sticky feeling on skin. *Hyarulonic acid* and *sodium pyrrolidone carboxylic acid* (PCA), which are humectants, may be used in addition to glycerin to decrease stickiness. It should be noted that application of a humectant alone can increase TEWL. For example, glycerin (glycerol) can increase TEWL by 29 percent. Thus, a humectant agent is usually combined with an occlusive ingredient, when used as a moisturizer.

Metals and botanical extracts are sometimes added in the moisturizers for their anti-inflammatory properties. Ginkgo biloba, green tea, aloe vera, allantoin, and licochalcone are botanical anti-inflammatory agents that are commonly used in the current market. The concentration of aloe vera should be at least 10 percent in order to have a moisturizing effect.Witch hazel is commonly used as an astringent in people with oily skin. Its high tannin content obtained by steam distillation of the plant may cause astringent action. Hamamelis ointments, known as witch hazel ointments, are used as acne cosmeceuticals. Currently, there are many metals, such as zinc, copper, selenium, aluminium, and strontium, that are used in cosmeceuticals. Well-established scientific data support the anti-inflammatory and wound healing benefits of zinc.

Anti-acne medications, including salicylic acid, benzoyl peroxide, and retinol, are commonly added to moisturizers

1. Retinol

Vitamin A derivatives, known as retinoids, are used in the treatment of acne. A variety of OTC retinoids exist that may be helpful in acne. These retinoids include retinol and retinaldehyde. Retinol can be absorbed by keratinocytes and reversibly oxidized into retinaldehyde. Retinaldehyde is irreversibly converted into all-trans retinoic acid, known as tretinoin, a potent prescription retinoid. Retinol has been shown to be twenty times less potent than topical tretinoin but exhibits greater penetration than tretinoin.

2. Tea Tree Oil

Another OTC topical nonmonographed agent used in botanical products for acne-prone skin is tea tree oil. Tea tree oil, obtained from the Australian tree *Melaleuca alternifolia*, contains several antimicrobial substances including: Terpinen-4-ol, alpha-terpineol, and alpha-pinene. The antibacterial activity of 10% tea tree oil has been shown against

Staphylococcus aureus, including methicillin-resistant *Staphylococcus aureus* (MRSA), without resistance. Lower concentrations, however, have demonstrated bacterial resistance. Tea tree oil has been found to be as effective in the treatment of acne as 5% benzoyl peroxide based on a reduction in comedones and inflammatory acne lesions; however, the onset of action was slower for tea tree oil [Bassett IB, 1990]. However, tea tree oil is a known cause of allergic contact dermatitis. An Italian study of 725 subjects patch tested with undiluted, 1%, and 0.1% tea tree oil found that 6% of subjects experienced a positive reaction to undiluted tea tree oil, 1 subject experience an allergic reaction to 1% tea tree oil, and no subjects experienced a reaction to the 0.1% dilution [Lisi P, 2000]. Thus, the incidence of allergic reactions to tea tree oil is concentration dependent.

In my practice I have noticed numerous cases of photosensitivity with tea tree oil. In fact a leading anti acne medication that contained clindamycin, aloe vera, and nicotinamide had tea tree oil and numerous patients had acute erythema and burning , which disappeared on using a identical combination without tea tree oil!

3. Miscellaneous Acne Ingredients

An ingredient of some interest in moisturizers for acne-prone skin is zinc. Zinc has been used in topical moisturizer formulations, since zinc salts are bacteriostatic to *P. acnes.*

A study by Dreno et al. demonstrated that zinc salts in the culture media of *P. acnes* prevented the development of organisms resistant to erythromycin. Since many *P. acnes* organisms are resistant to topical erythromycin, which has been largely replaced by topical clindamycin, this may be an important mechanism for preventing bacterial resistance. Another miscellaneous acne moisturizer ingredient is nicotinamide. Topical nicotinamide 4% was shown to be comparable to clindamycin gel 1% in the treatment of moderate acne [Shalita AR].

Surprisingly in India, formulations of clindamycin have in addition nicotinamide, which makes a little sense as their effect is comparable and not additive!

COSMETICS

The use of cosmetics like foundations, facial creams, anti-ageing creams, night creams and fairness creams are a major issue as most of them actually cause acne cosmetics. It is important that acne patients avoid contact with comedogenic ingredients [Draelos ZD, 2001]. Another issue is the role of our tropical weather, as in summer most acne patients have a flares of acne.

Patients with acne may wish to use facial foundations to camouflage acne lesions and aid in oil absorption. A facial foundation is a pigmented moisturizer applied over the entire face after cleansing. It contains iron oxide and zinc oxide to pigment the skin with a semitranslucent layer. Acne patients generally do best with an oil-free or low oil facial foundation. The facial foundation can be masked by dusting a loose pigmented powder on top to increase coverage, which is the ability of the cosmetic to camouage the skin, and also improve oil control. Most facial powders contain talc and kaolin, excellent oil absorbers, accompanied by iron oxide, the brown pigment that can be adjusted to match the patient's skin colour.

CONCLUSIONS

Most of the advice that we give to patients is countered by the ever increasing and persuasive MCG industry which through various ways, entice to try out products, most of which are comedogenic. Most of the so-called antiageing creams and moisturizers to an extent actually cause acne.

I follow a simple principle of advising a gel-based moisturizer and a mat finish sunscreen, if required. Minimising the use and time of application of retinoids and BPO can obviate the need of adjunctive cosmetics. The new microsphere formulations of retinoids and BPO are an attempt to minimize irritation and are ideal for Indian skin types. I follow the "less is more" dictum, thus the lesser cosmetics patients use the better their intrinsic skin, as in India, probably more acne is caused by the cosmetic industry than without!

REFERENCES

1. Bassett IB, Pannowitz DL. Barnetson RS A comparative study of tea-tree oil versus benzoyl peroxide in the treatment of acne. Med J Aust. 1990; 153(8):455–8.
2. Bojar RA, Cunliffe WJ, Holland KT. Short-term treatment of acne vulgaris with benzoyl peroxide: effects on the surface and follicular cutaneous microflora. Br J Dermatol. 1995; 132:204–8.
3. Chen T, Appa Y. Over-the-Counter Acne Medications. In: Draelos ZD, Thaman LA, editors. Cosmetic Formulations of Skin Care Products. New York: Taylor and Francis; 2006. p. 251–71.
4. Del Rosso JQ. Moisturizers: Function, formulation and clinical applications. In: Draelos Z, Dover JS, Alam M, editors. Cosmeceuticals. 2nd ed. China: Saunders Elsevier; 2009. pp. 97–102.
5. Draelos ZD. Cosmetics in acne and rosacea. Semin Cutan Med Surg. 2001; 20(3):209–14.

6. Dreno B, Trossaert M, Boiteau HL, Litoux P. Zinc salts effects on granulocyte zinc concentration and chemotaxis in acne patients. Acta Derm Venereol. 1992; 72(4):250–2.

7. Eady EA, Burke BM, Pulling K, Cunliffe WJ. The benefit of 2% salicylic acid lotion in acne. J Dermatol Therapy. 1996; 7:93–6.

8. Gupta AK, Nicol K, Gupta AK, Nicol K. The use of sulfur in dermatology. Journal of Drugs in Dermatology. 2004; 3(4):427–31.

9. Laquieze S, Czernielewski J, Rueda MJ. Beneficial effect of a moisturizing cream as adjunctive treatment to oral isotretinoin or topical tretinoin in the management of acne. J Drugs Dermatol. 2006; 5:985–990.

10. Leyden JJ, Wortzman M, Baldwin EK. Antibiotic-resistant Propionibacterium acnes suppressed by a benzoyl peroxide cleanser 6%. Cutis. 2008; 82(6):417–21.

11. Leyden JJ, Del Rosso JQ. The effect of benzoyl peroxide 9.8% emollient foam on reduction of Propionibacterium acnes on the back using a short contact therapy approach. J Drugs Dermatol. 2012 Jul; 11(7):830–3.

12. Leyden JJ. The effect of benzoyl peroxide 6% wash on antibiotic-resistant propionibacterium acnes. Poster presented at: 31st Hawaii Dermatology Seminar; March 3–9, 2007; Wailea, Maui, Hawaii.

13. Lin AN, Reimer RJ, Carter DM. Sulfur revisited. J Amer Acad Dermatol. 1988; 18(3):553–8.

14. Lisi P, Melingi L, Pigatto P, Ayala F, Suppa F, Foti C, Angelini G. Prevalenza della sensibilizzazione all'olio exxenziale di Melaleuca. Ann Ital Dermatol Allergol. 2000; 54:141–4.

15. Mills OH, Kligman AM. Evaluation of abrasives in acne therapy. Cutis. 1979; 23:704–5.

16. Shalita AR, Smith JG, Parish LC, Sofman MS, Chalker DK. Topical nicotinamide compared with clindamycin gel in the treatment of inflammatory acne vulgaris. Int J Dermatol. 1999; 34(6):434–7.

VI. ACNE SCARS: SURGICAL AND COSMETIC TREATMENTS

INTRODUCTION

Acne is a common, chronic, inflammatory disorder in practice. It involves the pilosebaceous follicles and occurs predominantly on the face in teenagers and young adults. It is increasingly being seen in older adults beyond 25 years of age, which is termed adult acne.

Unfortunately facial scarring following acne may occur early in the disease affecting up to 95% of patients. Acne scars lead to major psychological stress in young patients. The degree of scarring depends on the severity of acne, inappropriate management and delay in treatment. Therefore, it is important for all practitioners to correctly treat acne early and adequately in order to prevent permanent scars.

TYPES OF ACNE SCARS

Post-acne scars are polymorphic and different types of scars may coexist in the same patient.

They are classified into various types, depending on the colour, depth and contour (Table 4.9 and Fig. 4.6).

Clinical Features

Ice pick scars are small scars (1–2 mm), have wide mouths and taper down to a single point at the bottom in the dermis (Fig. 4.6c). Rolling scars are, broad, shallow scars best appreciated in indirect light. They

Table 4.9 *Types of acne scars*

Macular–flat scars

- Erythematous (persistent reddish scars) (Fig. 4.6a)
- Hyperpigmented (persistent dark scars) (Fig. 4.6b)

Atrophic–depressed scars

- Icepick (Fig. 4.6d)
- Rolling (Fig. 4.6d)
- Boxcar (Fig. 4.6c)

Elevated–raised scars

- Hypertrophic (Fig. 4.6e)
- Keloidal (Fig. 4.6e)
- Papular (Fig. 4.6f)
- Bridging scars and sinus tracts

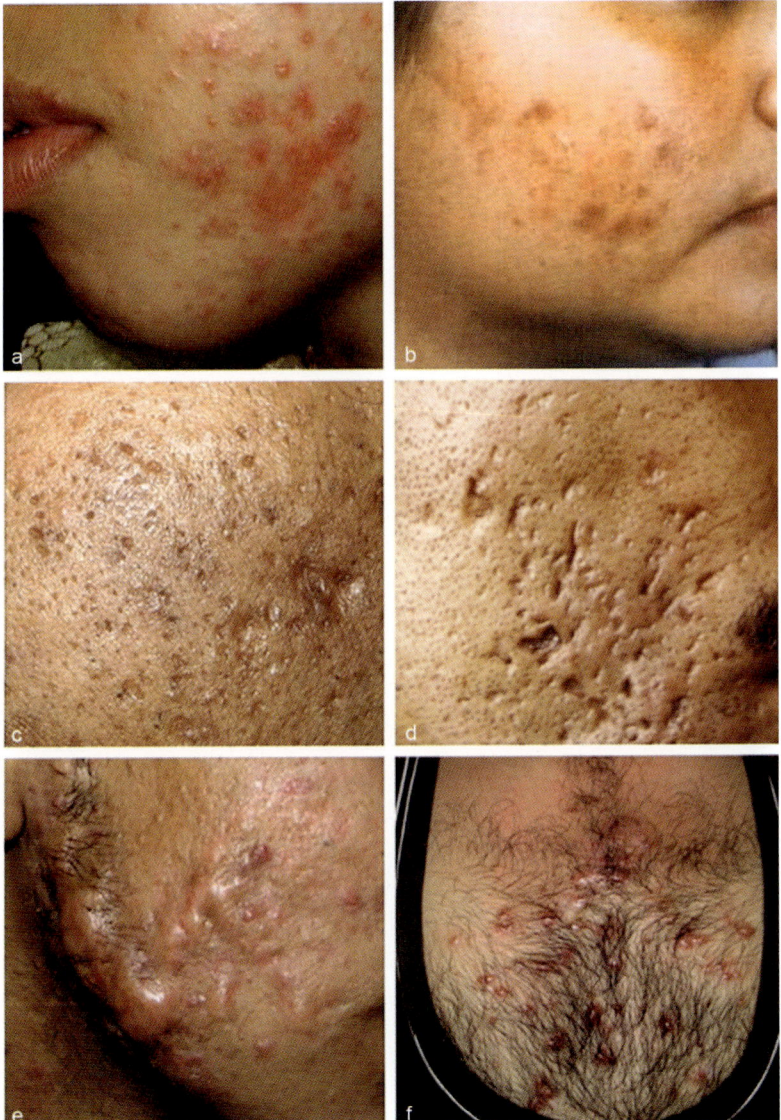

Fig. 4.6: Types of acne scars: (a) Macular erythematous scars, (b) macular hyperpigmented scars, (c) atropic boxcar scars, (d) atrophic icepick and rolling scars, (e) hypertophic scars (keloidal), (f) hypertophic scars (papular scars)

occur due to dermal tethering of almost normal looking skin. Boxcar scars are deep, punched out, round or oval, shaped scars, having similar width at the surface and the base with vertical walls.

Hypertrophic scars usually develop on the trunk and the lower half of the face. Keloids may also be a complication of acne; the basic difference between hypertrophic scars and keloids is that the former does not extend beyond the area of original inflammation, whereas keloids do.

Management

Since different types of scars often coexist in the same patient, there is no single best treatment and multiple treatment modalities are required. Therefore, treating acne scars is a real challenge.

Counseling

Before starting treatment it is important to counsel the patient as expectations are very high from any procedure. Judge the motivation of the patient and bring down expectations of the media-hyped patient. Explain the nature of treatment and downplay the expected degree of improvement. Discuss time taken for recovery of normal skin, possible side-effects and pigmentary changes that may occur. Patient education regarding avoidance of practices like squeezing and manipulating lesions is important.

ASSESSMENT OF THE PATIENT AND PRE-TREATMENT

Assess if there is a keloidal tendency or family history of keloids. Be careful if there is a history of herpes simplex or recent isotretinoin treatment in the last six months, assess the degree of sun exposure of the patient as an outdoor occupation with prolonged exposure to the sun increases the risk of complications. *Examine* the activity of acne, type of acne scars, severity and overall appearance of the patient. *Document* the treatment taken, take an informed consent and keep a photographic record before treatment. *Priming is preparation of the skin to avoid complications.* This should be done at least two to four weeks before any procedure. Avoiding sun exposure and sunscreens use is important. Topical tretinoin 0.25–0.05%, 2–4% hydroquinone, 0.75–2% kojic acid, glycolic acid 6–12% can be used in the evening.

TREATMENT

Treatment of acne scars is mainly procedural. Various over the counter creams that are advertised for scars will not help most scars and may be beneficial only for early flat scars.

There are various procedures that can be used (Table 4.10).

The choice of the procedure depends on the severity and the type of scars and they can be combined to give optimum results.

Table 4.10 *Procedures for acne scars*

Noninvasive
- Topical therapy
- Nonablative lasers, radiofrequency and light therapy
- Silicon gels and sheets

Minimally invasive
- Subcision
- Chemical peeling
- Microneedling
- Microdermabrasion
- TCA CROSS technique
- Fillers
- Fractional CO_2 or Erbium YAG laser

Invasive
- Punch excision techniques
- Laser resurfacing
- Scar excision
- Dermabrasion

Macular pigmented scars: Topical hypopigmenting agents like 4% hydroquinone, 10% glycolic acid, 20% azelaic acid, 2% kojic acid are useful for persistent pigmented scars. Chemical peeling with 20–50% salicylic acid or glycolic acid 35–70% is effective for scars that do not respond or to quicken the response (Fig. 4.7).

Icepick scars: They are the most difficult to treat. Subcision, TCA CROSS technique, punch excision techniques are utilized in combination followed by microneedling or resurfacing with lasers (Fig. 4.8).

Rolling scars: Subcision, followed by microneedling or fillers, hyaluronic acid (Restylane, Perlane), acrylamide gel (Esthelis, Aquamid) or autologous fat are useful techniques. These can be followed by laser resurfacing.

Boxcar scars: Punch excision followed by suturing or grafting is performed initially followed by resurfacing by lasers (Fig. 4.9).

Papular scars: Intralesional radiofrequency or Er:YAG laser.

Hypertrophic scars: Intralesional corticosteroids (triamcinolone acetonide) 10 mg/ml (Fig. 4.10).

Keloidal scars: Debulking with radiofrequency surgery followed immediately with intralesional triamcinolone acetonide 20–40 mg/ml or 5-fluorouracil 50 mg/ml.

Multiple sinus tracts: Excision of tracts, evacuate contents, excise scarred tissue and suture along RSTL.

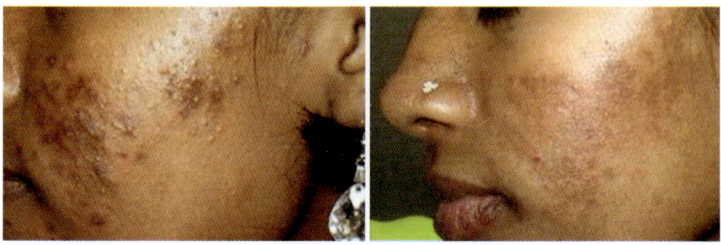

Fig. 4.7: Macular hyperpigmented scars treated with salicylic acid chemical peels

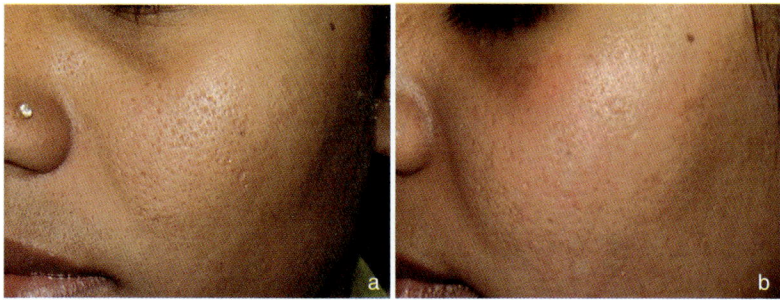

Fig. 4.8: Icepick scars: (a) before treatment, (b) after treatment

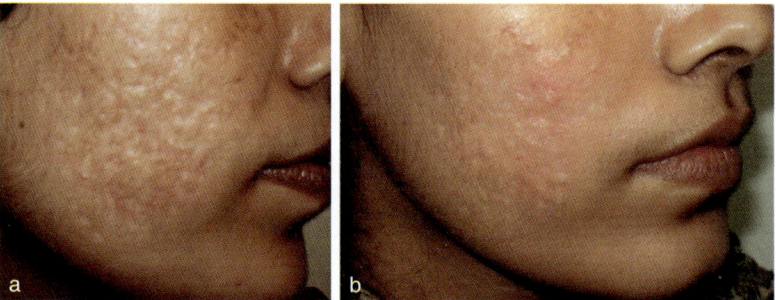

Fig. 4.9: Rolling scars treated with subcision and microneedling: (a) before treatment, (b) after treatment

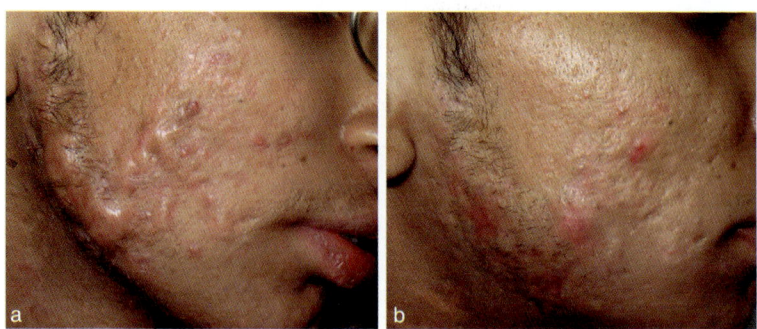

Fig. 4.10: Hypertrophic scars treated with intralesional steroids: (a) before treatment, (b) after treatment

LASERS FOR ACNE SCARS

Though lasers are widely advertised as the magic wand for all scars, they are not useful for all scars and all skin types. Lasers which ablate the skin have a higher incidence of side effects especially in darker skin types. Hence fractional CO_2 or fractional Erbium YAG lasers are safer, whereas results are mild and slow with nonablative lasers (Figs 4.11 and 4.12). Fractional lasers have a major advantage over the previous conventional ablative methods and these should be

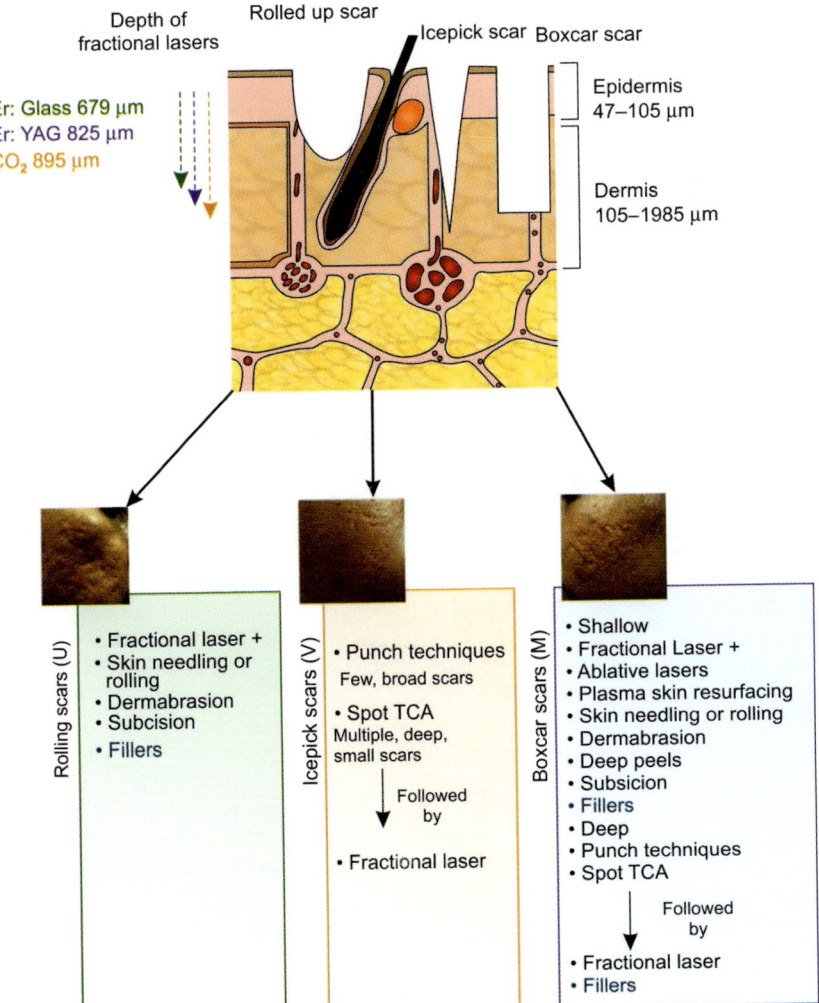

Fig. 4.11: A depiction of the types of scars with the ideal method of treatment for each type of scars. The figure above depicts the depth of the scars, with depth of the fractional lasers. (Source: Sardana K, *Lasers in Dermatological Practice*, 2015, Jaypee Pub)

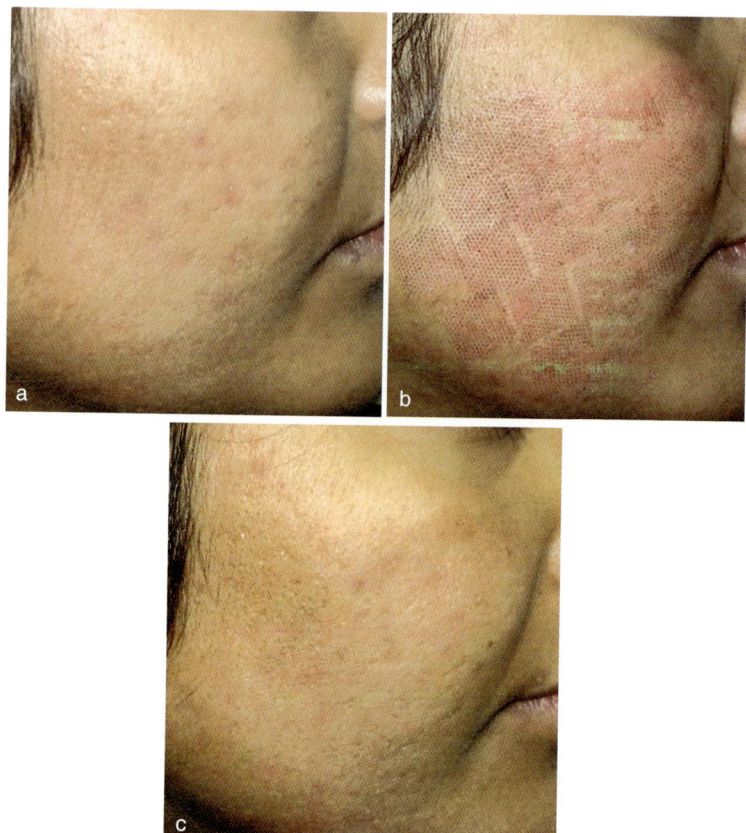

Fig. 4.12: (a) Treatment with fractional CO_2 laser, before treatment, (b) immediately following treatment with fractional CO_2 laser, (c) one week after treatment

preferentially used because of their quicker recovery time, favourable side effect profile and good clinical outcomes.

Complications

If not done by trained qualified physicians, complications can occur frequently. Hyperpigmentation, that is, excessive darkening, hypopigmentation or spotty lighter spots, persistent erythema and worsening of scars can occur. The commonest complication is patient dissatisfaction as most patients expect miracles and a flawless skin, which is difficult to achieve.

CONCLUSION

The treatment of acne scars requires a multimodality approach by a trained physician. An array of treatment options are available, but none is best or singly or wholly effective. Treatments should be individualized according to the type and severity of scars and the patient skin type. The patient must be made to understand that the main goal of treatment is to achieve improvement as much as possible instead of perfection. However, it is important for practitioners to be aware of the various treatment modalities available so that they can guide the patients accordingly. Early and superficial scars are easier to treat than deep and severe scars. Hence prevention of scars is important and the practitioner must treat acne correctly and refer when required.

VII. DIET AND ACNE

The current status of the relation between diet and acne is unclear and under debate. On one hand, the American Academy of Dermatology (AAD) published recommendations [Strauss et al., 2007] in 2007 suggesting that caloric restriction has no benefit in the treatment of acne and that there is insufficient evidence to link the consumption of certain "food enemies" to acne (http://www. skincarephysicians. com. acnenet acne_and_diet. html). On the other hand, recent clinical studies have suggested a rather close relation between diet and acne [Smith et al., 2007].

We will present the data at hand that suggest that certain nutrients play a role in acne. Also the argument linking high glycaemic diet with acne, hinges on the role of insulin, and may be relevant to the persistence of acne. But the lack of acne in diabetics is still inexplicable and is an argument against the insulin hypothesis.

VITAMIN A

Oral administration of isotretinoin (13-cis-retinoic acid) and topical application of its isomers and natural retinoids (e.g. tretinoin) are used as anti-acne therapies. 13-cis-retinoic acid (RA) is the only drug that targets all four pathogenic factors of acne and is the most efficient so far in regard to sebum suppression. 13-cis-RA is a retinoid that potentially derives from the metabolism of vitamin A. Although several websites state that it is found in small quantities naturally in the body without citing a reference [Vahlquist, 1999], we know that at least the natural isomers of RA also affect the disease.

The superlative effect of isotretinoin, a vitamin A derivative, is a good argument of the role of nutrients in acne, though the quantity required of oral Vitamin A is extremely high to individually effect a treatment response.

EFA

There are also two fatty acids in our body that are essential and cannot be synthesized by human cells: linoleic acid (18:2, D9,12) and linolenic acid (18:2, D9,12,15) (LA). These are important nutrients that need to be obtained from the diet, which is why they are referred to as essential fatty acids. These two essential nutrients are precursors to the omega-6 (γ-linoleic acid) and omega-3 fatty acid (α-linolenic acid) families, respectively, a family of metabolites that are involved in numerous important physiological processes, including inflammation. Consequently we could safely assume that the absence of these important nutrients from our diet could have important implications for both acne and our overall health.

Numerous studies have revealed that clinical imbalances of specific essential fatty acids are associated with a variety of skin problems, such as dry, itchy, scaly skin, which is a hallmark sign of fatty acid deficiency. More relevant to this is a publication that suggested that the sebum of acne patients is relatively deficient in linoleic acid [Downing et al., 1986].

A recent nutritional clinical study [De Spirt et al., 2009] in two groups of women who consumed flaxseed (omega-3 fatty acid) or borage oil (omega-6) for 12 weeks revealed that the daily ingestion of 2.2 g total fatty acids with *alpha*-linolenic acid and linoleic acid as major constituents in the *flaxseed oil* group and linoleic and *gamma*-linolenic acid in the borage oil group, demonstrated skin benefits. Skin irritation, changes in skin reddening, and blood flow were diminished in both groups compared to the placebo group, providing evidence that skin properties can be modulated by intervention with dietary fats.

The fact that Western diets are often deficient in the longer-chain omega-3 FA and their precursor alpha-LA raises an additional issue for this discussion. It is known that the ratio of omega-6 to omega-3 fatty acids in a typical western diet ranges from about 10:1 to 20:1 versus a ratio of 3:1–1:1 in a non-Western diet or in primitive, non-industrialized populations. These findings were the foundation for population studies that revealed that non-Western diets correlated with the absence of acne [Cordain et al., 2002]. A number of studies have suggested that inflammatory markers correlate with an increase of the omega-6/omega-3 ratio [Kris-Etherton et al., 2000]. The *omega-6* fatty acids are thought to induce more *proinflammatory* mediators and have been associated with the development of inflammatory acne [Zouboulis, 2001]. On the other hand, intake of high levels of *omega-3* fatty acids is linked with decreases in inflammatory factors [James et al., 2000]. In addition, there are epidemiological studies demonstrating that increasing the intake of *omega-3* fatty acids through a diet rich in seafood results in lower rates of inflammatory disease [Kris-Etherton et al., 2000].

Thus in essence diets rich in fresh vegetables, fish, flaxseed oil, DHA/EPA , which are all rich in omega-3 EFA will have a salutary effect on acne.

ESSENTIAL ELEMENTS

Another class of nutrients that derives from the diet includes minerals such as zinc, copper, selenium, and iron, which known to influence anti-inflammatory and proinflammatory enzymes (e.g. desaturases and lipoxygenases). We have shown the superlative effects of zinc in acne, specially with the methionine based zinc [Sardana K].

HIGH GLYCEMIC DIET

It has been reported that people living in the Kitavan Islands (off the coast of Papua New Guinea) and the Aché hunter-gathers of Paraguay do not suffer from acne and that it is associated with their low-glycemic diet, consisting mainly of fresh vegetables, fruits, and lean proteins [Cordain, et al. 2002].

This conclusion is in agreement with the latest studies [Smith, et al. 2007] on low-glycemic diets (discussed later). In brief, one prospective cohort study [Smith, et al. 2007] found a valid association between high-glycemic-index foods and longer acne duration, whereas low-glycemic-index diet had a reduced acne risk. The work of Smith et al (2007) focused on the glycemic load, insulin sensitivity, hormonal mediators, and acne. The investigators reported that foods with a high glycemic index contribute to acne by elevating serum insulin concentrations (which may stimulate sebocyte proliferation and sebum production), suppress SHBG concentrations, and raise androgen concentrations. On the contrary, low glycemic index foods increased SHBG and reduced androgen levels, which is important because high SHBG levels were associated with less acne severity.

Recently, Spencer et al. (2009) and Bowe et al (2010) summarized 27 relevant studies: 21 were observational, and 6 were clinical trials and concluded that although there is compelling evidence for the association of acne and high-glycemic-load diets, there is weak evidence for an association between dairy product ingestion and acne.

CONCLUSION

There are still questions as why not all obese individuals have long-term acne as most people who are obese demonstrate insulin resistance. In addition, if insulin resistance is associated with acne, everyone who suffers from diabetes type 2 would be expected to have acne. Nevertheless, a high glycemic load seems to be associated with the occurrence of acne, and a recommendation for a low-glycemic load diet cannot harm the affected population. How bad could it be when such a diet, which includes a variety of fruits and vegetables, lean protein, and healthy fats, can also protect against cardiovascular disease, type 2 diabetes, metabolic syndrome, and even obesity?

Thus it is a good common sense advise to tell patients to avoid processed foods, cheese, simple carbohydrates and increase the intake of EFA of the omega-3 kind. I do this and whether national recommendations differ, are not relevant as if a clinician can make a difference in the eating patterns of patients a lot more good than harm is done!

REFERENCES

1. Bowe WP, Joshi SS, Shalita AR. Diet and acne. J Am Acad Dermatol. 2010; 63(1):124–41. Epub 2010 Mar 24. Review.

2. Cordain L, Lindeberg S, Hurtado M, Hill K, Eaton SB, Brand-Miller J. Acne vulgaris: a disease of western civilization. Arch Dermatol. 2002; 138(12):1584–90.

3. Downing DT, Stewart ME, Wertz PW, Strauss JS. Essential fatty acids and acne. J Am Acad Dermatol. 1986; 14(2 Pt 1):221–5.

4. James MJ, Gibson RA, Cleland LG. Dietary polyunsaturated fatty acids and inflammatory mediator production. Am J Clin Nutr. 2000; 71(1 Suppl):343S–8. Review.

5. Kris-Etherton PM, Taylor DS, Yu-Poth S, Huth P, Moriarty K, Fishell V, et al. Polyunsaturated fatty acids in the food chain in the united states. Am J Clin Nutr. 2000; 71(1 Suppl):179S–88. Review.

6. Smith RN, Mann NJ, Braue A, et al. The effect of a high-protein, low glycemic-load diet versus a conventional, high glycemic-load diet on biochemical parameters associated with acne vulgaris: a randomized, investigator-masked, controlled trial. J Am Acad Dermatol. 2007; 57:247–56.

7. Smith RN, Mann NJ, Braue A, et al. The effect of a high-protein, low glycemic-load diet versus a conventional, high glycemic-load diet on biochemical parameters associated with acne vulgaris: a randomized, investigator-masked, controlled trial. J Am Acad Dermatol. 2007b; 57:247–56.

8. Spencer EH, Ferdowsian HR, Barnard ND. Diet and acne: a review of the evidence. Int J Dermatol. 2009; 48(4):339–47. Review.

9. Strauss JS, Krowchuk DP, Leyden JJ, Lucky AW, Shalita AR, Siegfried EC, et al. American Academy of Dermatology/American Academy of Dermatology Association. Guidelines of care for acne vulgaris management. J Am Acad Dermatol. 2007; 56(4):651–63. Epub 2007 Feb 5. Review.

10. Vahlquist A. What are natural retinoids? Dermatology. 1999;199 Suppl 1:3–11. Review.

11. Zouboulis CC. Is acne vulgaris a genuine inflammatory disease? Dermatology. 2001; 203(4):277–9.

5

Guidelines of Treatment

I. CNE IN ADULTS

Acne is now considered a chronic disease and hence its management is divided into induction and maintenance phase. Early and aggressive treatment of acne is warranted as it leads to early resolution of lesions and reduces the sequelae of both physical and emotional scarring. To preserve the success of initial treatment and to prevent frequent relapses, maintenance therapy is important in the treatment of acne. Management of acne should be based on multifactorial considerations which are beyond the clinically determined acne severity and should incorporate patient-reported impact, gender, skin sensitivity and phototype. As the most recent guideline is the European evidence based guidelines for treatment of acne, this will be followed in this chapter as shown in Table 5.1 (Nast A et al, 2012).

TREATMENT OF COMEDONAL ACNE

1. Topical therapy is generally preferred over systemic therapy for the treatment of comedonal acne due to its usually mild to moderate presentation.

2. Due to the lack of direct evidence for the treatment of comedonal acne, no treatment is recommended as a high strength recommendation (Table 5.1).

3. Topical *retinoids, benzoyl peroxide (BPO) and azelaic acid* are found to have best efficacies for the treatment of comedonal acne.

4. Efficacy of various agents in the treatment of comedonal acne:

   a. *Efficacy of topical agents used as monotherapy:* There are conflicting results from the studies comparing the efficacy of topical retinoids in the treatment of non-inflammatory lesions

98

Table 5.1 *Therapeutic recommendations for treatment of acne**

	Comedonal acne	Mild-moderate papulopustular acne	Severe papulopustular or moderate	Severe nodular or conglobate acne§ nodular acne
High strength of recommendation	None	Adapalene + BPO (fc) or BPO + clindamycin (fc) Clindamycin should be limited for 3 months	Oral isotretinoin	Oral isotretinoin (Expert opinion: For the initial treatment phase with isotretinoin a combination with oral corticosteroids treatment can be considered in conglobate acne)
Medium strength of recommendation	Topical retinoids (adapalene to be preferred over tretinoin or isotretinoin)	Azelaic acid or BPO or Topical retinoid. (adapalene to be preferred to tretinoin or isotretinoin) In case of widespread disease/ moderate severity use combination of systemic antibiotic + adapalene	Systemic antibiotics + Adapalene/ Azelaic acid/ Adapalene-BPO (fc) (doxycycline or lymecycline limited to treatment period of 3 months)	Systemic antibiotics (doxycycline or lymecycline) + Azelaic acid

(*Contd.*)

Table 5.1 *Therapeutic recommendations for treatment of acne* (Contd.)*

	Comedonal acne	Mild-moderate papulopustular acne	Severe papulopustular or moderate nodular acne	Severe nodular or conglobate acne[§]
Low strength of recommendation	Azelaic acid *or* BPO	Blue light *or* Oral zinc *or* Topical erythromycin + isotretinoin (fc) *or* Topical erythromycin + tretinoin (fc) *or* Systemic antibiotics* (doxycycline or lymecycline) + BPO *or* Systemic antibiotics* (doxycycline or lymecycline) + azelaic acid *or* Systemic antibiotics* (doxycycline or lymecycline) + adapalene + BPO (fc)	Systemic antibiotics (doxycycline or lymecycline) + BPO	Systemic antibiotics (doxycycline or lymecycline) + BPO/ Adapalene adapalene-BPO (fc)

(Contd.)

Table 5.1 *Therapeutic recommendations for treatment of acne* (Contd.)*

	Comedonal acne	Mild-moderate papulopustular acne	Severe papulopustular or moderate nodular acne	Severe nodular or conglobate acne§
Negative recommendation	Topical antibiotics, hormonal antiandrogens, systemic antibiotics, systemic isotretinoin and/or artificial ultraviolet radiation are not recommended	Topical antibiotics monotherapy, artificial UV radiation, erythromycin + zinc (fc), systemic antibiotics oral isotretinoin or hormonal antiandrogens are not recommended	Artificial UV radiation or monotherapy with single or combined topical agents/oral antibiotics/ oral anti-androgens/ visible light are not recommended	Artificial UV radiation sources or monotherapy with topical agents/oral antibiotics/ oral anti-androgens/ visible light are not recommended
Open recommendation	Recommendation for or against visible light as monotherapy, lasers with visible wavelengths, lasers with infrared wavelengths, IPL and PDT for the treatment of comedonal acne cannot be made at present	No recommendation at present either for or against the use of red light, IPL, laser or PDT	Recommendation for or against IPL, laser and PDT cannot be made at present	No recommendation at present either for or against the use of IPL, laser or PDT

(Contd.)

Table 5.1 *Therapeutic recommendations for treatment of acne* (Contd.)*

	Comedonal acne	Mild-moderate papulopustular acne	Severe papulopustular or moderate nodular acne	Severe nodular or conglobate acne[§]
Alternatives for female patients	—	—	Hormonal antiandrogens + topical treatment or Hormonal antiandrogens + systemic antibiotics (doxycycline or lymecycline limited to treatment period of 3 months)	Hormonal antiandrogens + systemic antibiotics (doxycycline or lymecycline limited to treatment period of 3 months)

*In case of more widespread disease or moderate severity, initiation of a systemic therapy can be recommended.
§Systemic treatment with corticosteroids can be considered.
fc: fixed combination, BPO: benzoyl peroxide, UV: ultraviolet, IPL: intense pulsed light, PDT: photodynamic therapy.

(NIL) of acne. The efficacy of adapalene against the NIL was found to be *comparable*, if not superior to tretinoin (Nyirady et al, 2001). The efficacy of isotretinoin was found to be *comparable* to adapalene (Ioannides et al, 2002) and superior to tretinoin (Dominguez, 1998). The efficacy of BPO was *comparable* to adapalene and isotretinoin, and comparable-to-superior to tretinoin.

The efficacy of azelaic acid was *comparable* to adapalene and *inferior* to both BPO and tretinoin. The efficacy of monotherapy with antibiotics like clindamycin and erythromycin was found to be *inferior* to BPO, isotretinoin, tretinoin and azelaic acid.

b. *Efficacy of topical combination therapy*: The efficacy of fixed dose combination (FDC) of BPO and adapalene was comparable-to-superior to either of the agents used as monotherapy for the treatment of NIL although there was a trend for the deterioration in the *tolerability* profile (Korkut and Piskin, 2005). The efficacy of fixed dose combination of clindamycin and BPO was comparable to BPO and adapalene and superior to clindamycin. Fixed dose combinations of clindamycin-BPO and adapalene-BPO were found to be *comparable* to each other.

5. Though only indirect data is available, patients showed preference for adapalene amongst the topical retinoids (Kellett et al, 2006).

6. The pathophysiology of comedone formation favours the use of topical retinoids.

7. Topical retinoids and BPO have comparable tolerability profile. Azelaic acid was found to have superior *tolerability/safety* profile than tretinoin (Katsambas et al, 1989).

8. At present, no recommendation can be made for or against the use of lasers and light sources for the treatment of comedonal acne due to lack of experience, clinical trials and standard protocols.

Summary

There are three issues of concern: efficacy, tolerability and resistance profile. Thus in Indian skin that is predisposed to irritation and post-inflammatory hyperpigmentation (PIH) agents that can minimise irritation while being effective are important. Thus adapalene, micronized tretinoin, FDC that are gentle and azelaic acid is ideal. Plain BPO may be an issue in some patients, so FDC with clindamycin are better. Adapalene/BPO can cause marked irritation in some patients, but if tolerated is the ideal FDC.

TREATMENT OF PAPULOPUSTULAR ACNE

1. Severe papulopustular or moderate nodular acne should be treated with **systemic therapy** as they increase the efficacy, adherence and patient satisfaction. Addition of topical agents can further enhance the efficacy (Table 5.1).

2. There is high strength of recommendation for oral isotretinoin in the management of severe papulopustular acne owing to its high efficacy seen in clinical practise.

3. The efficacy of various agents in the treatment of papulopustular acne are:

   a. *Efficacy of topical therapy:* Fixed dose combination of BPO with adapalene and BPO with clindamycin have shown *highest* efficacies against the inflammatory lesions (IL) of acne as compared to topical monotherapies and their efficacies are comparable to each other (Zouboulis et al, 2009). The efficacy of combination of BPO and adapalene against the IL of acne was comparable-to-superior to monotherapy with BPO and superior to monotherapy with adapalene (Gollnick et al, 2009). The combination of clindamycin and BPO has *superior* efficacy than either agents used as monotherapy (Ellis et al, 2001).

b. *The efficacy of topical versus systemic therapy*: Switching from monotherapy with topical agent to monotherapy with systemic antibiotics does not increase the efficacy. However, combination of systemic antibiotic *with* a topical agent shows a trend towards *increased efficacy* as compared to systemic antibiotic used alone.

Systemic isotretinoin has *comparable* efficacy to combination of minocycline and azelaic acid on the IL of acne (Gollnick, 2001), however, isotretinoin has a more rapid onset of action. The efficacy of systemic isotretinoin was also superior to combination of tetracycline plus adapalene. Lymecycline and adapalene combination was superior to monotherapy with lymecycline. Combination of doxycycline and adapalene showed a trend towards superior efficacy than monotherapy with doxycycline.

c. Amongst the anti-androgens, ethinyloestradiol and cyproteronacetate have shown superior efficacy than ethinyloestradiol and levonorgestrel (EE-LG) and comparable efficacy to ethinyloestradiol and desogestrel. The efficacy of ethinyloestradiol and drospirenone and ethinyloestradiol and norgestimate is comparable. There is scarce and conflicting evidence comparing systemic antibiotics with oral contraceptives (Table 5.2).

4. Amongst light and laser therapy, only blue light has been found to have superior efficacy to placebo against inflammatory and total lesions of acne. The evidence is conflicting regarding the efficacy of red light in acne and insufficient regarding the efficacy of all other

Table 5.2 *Efficacy of contraceptives vs. systemic antibiotics in papulopustular acne*

	Tetracycline(T) [level of evidence]	Minocycline(M) [level of evidence]
Ethinylestradiol and cyproteronacetate (EE-CPA)	EE-CPA > T	EE-CPA = M [3]
Etinylestradiol and cyproteronacetate + tetracycline	EE-CPA + T > T	X

EE-CPA: Ethinylestradiol and cyproteronacetate; M: minocycline; X: no evidence; T: tetracycline.

laser and light therapy as compared to placebo. There is lack of standardized treatment protocol for use of lasers and light in treating papulopustular acne.

5. Tolerability and safety profile of various agents used in the management of papulopustular acne are as follows:

a. *Topical agents used alone or in combinations*: *Azelaic acid* (15% or 20%) has superior safety and tolerability profile as compared to adapalene, tretinoin and 5% BPO. Adapalene has best safety and tolerability profile amongst topical retinoids followed by isotretinoin and tretinoin and trials have confirmed its preference amongst patients (LE 3). Owing to the best safety and tolerability profile of adapalene and comparable efficacy in the treatment of IL of acne amongst the retinoids, use of *adapalene* should be preferred to tretinoin and isotretinoin. BPO has comparable tolerability and safety profile as compared to topical retinoids, with lower concentration of BPO showing better tolerability and safety.

The combination of BPO and clindamycin has *superior* tolerability and safety profile to combination of BPO and adapalene. The safety and tolerability of BPO and clindamycin combination on the IL of acne was comparable to BPO monotherapy and inferior to clindamycin monotherapy. The safety and tolerability of combination of BPO and adapalene is inferior to BPO mono-therapy and inferior-to-comparable to adapalene monotherapy.

b. *Systemic and topical therapy*: Combination of *minocycline* and *azelaic acid* was more safe and tolerable as compared to oral isotretinoin. The safety and tolerability of doxycycline was comparable to combination of doxycycline-and-adapalene and doxycycline-adapalene-BPO combination. Lymecycline was more safe and tolerable than combination of lymecycline and adapalene.

6. *Doxycycline and lymecycline* should be preferred over minocycline and tetracycline due to less frequent and less severe drug reactions and superior practicability. The efficacies of all these four antibiotics are comparable to each other in the treatment of IL of acne and tetracycline shows a trend towards comparable-to-superior efficacy than clindamycin and erythromycin. No clear evidence is available at present regarding superior safety and tolerability of one antibiotic over the other; however, systemic review by Smith and Leyden found that the adverse effects were more common and severe with minocycline as compared to doxycycline (Smith, Leyden JJ, 2005). Garner et al reported the incidence of adverse drug reaction as 11.1% with minocycline, 13.1% with tetracycline or oxytetracycline and

6.1% with doxycycline (Garner et al, 2003). Adverse drug reactions are reported with all the antibiotics, but the reactions with doxycycline are easy to manage (sun protection for photosensitivity and increase intake of water for oesophagitis) as compared to those seen with minocycline (hypersensitivity, hepatic dysfunction, lupus like syndrome). Phototoxicity due to doxycycline depends upon the amount of sunlight and the dose of the drug taken. Phototoxicity is less common with lymecycline than doxycycline and the safety profile of lymecycline is comparable to tetracycline. Systemic clindamycin should be reserved for only treating severe infection and its use is *not* recommended routinely. Frequent administration of tetracycline makes it less practical in its use by patients.

7. Apart from the known molecular mechanism of resistance to *P. acnes* due to mutations in genes coding 23S and 16S rRNA, there are still many strains with unidentified mutations suggesting new mechanism of resistance in *P. acnes*. Combined resistance to clindamycin and erythromycin (91% in Spain) is more commonly seen as compared to tetracycline (26% in UK). Whereas the resistance caused by topical antibiotics is confined to the site of application, oral antibiotics can cause development of resistance in commensal flora at all body sites. Resistance is more commonly seen in patients with moderate-to-severe acne and in countries which have high outpatient sale of antibiotics. Since the resistance spreads by person-to-person contact, it is primarily the treating physicians and family and friends of the affected patient who are responsible for the diss-emination of resistance. Although there is data suggesting that the resistant strains may disappear after discontinuation of the antibiotic, there is also data suggesting persistence and rapid reactivation of stains even after discontinuation of antibiotics. The most likely effect of antibiotic resistance could be a poor therapeutic response and a few trials have proved the diminishing efficacy of topical erythromycin. In contrast there are also trials which show that there is no decrease in the efficacy of topical clindamycin and oral tetracycline in the past few decades. Due to emerging drug resistance, the indication and duration of systemic antibiotics should be limited and monotherapy with both topical and systemic antibiotics should be avoided. The physicians should minimize the spread of cross infection while examining the patient and BPO should be added to prevent development of antibiotic resistance.

8. There are no conclusive comparison on the safety and tolerability profile on comparison of anti-androgens and isotretinoin with other systemic agents.

SUMMARY

Systemic cyclines, isotretinoin with topical azelaic acid, adapalene or FDC is the simplest method to balance efficacy and tolerability.

Note that the use of macrolides is not advisable routinely as they predispose to resistance and are also used in many medical indications. Thus contrary to the indiscriminate use of azithromycin for acne, it has a little advantage over cyclines.

TREATMENT OF NODULAR AND CONGLOBATE ACNE

A summary of the treatment is given in Table 5.3 for quick reference:

1. The guidelines on the indication of oral isotretinoin in the management of acne by European Union directive states that "oral isotretinoin should only be used in severe acne, nodular and conglobate acne, that has or is not responding to appropriate antibiotics and topical therapy". This essentially means that oral isotretinoin cannot be used at all as a first line therapy. However, the European Evidence Based Guidelines for the treatment of acne supports and recommends the use of oral isotretinoin as the first drug of choice for the treatment of severe papulopustular, moderate-

Table 5.3 *Efficacy of therapies for nodular and conglobate acne*

	Systemic tetracycline (st) [level of evidence]	Systemic isotretinoin (si) [level of evidence]
Topical clindamycin (tc)	st > tc	X
Azelaic acid (aa)	aa = st	X
Systemic minocycline (sm)	X	si > sm
Systemic tetracycline (st)	X	si > st
Azelaic acid + mino-cycline(aa-m)	X	si = aa-m
Tetracycline + adapalene (t-a)	X	si = t-a
Isotretinoin + clindamycin + adapalene (i-c-a)	X	si = i-c-a

a: adapalene; aa: azelaic acid; c: clindamycin; i: isotretinoin; m: minocycline; X: no evidence; t: tetracycline.

to-severe nodular and conglobate acne due to its rapid reduction in inflammation seen in acne, prevention of clinical and psychological scarring, quick improvement in the quality of life and reduction in the risk of depression (Layton, 2001; Rubinow et al, 1987). The rate of relapse in acne is lowest with oral isotretinoin as compared to all other available therapies.

2. The efficacy of various agents used in the treatment of nodular and conglobate acne is shown in Table 5.3. Most of the studies used 0.5 mg/kg bodyweight of oral isotretinoin and showed a mean reduction of 70% in the nodular and conglobate acne. There was no additional benefit of adding topical clindamycin and adapalene to oral isotretinoin as compared to monotherapy with oral isotretinoin. The efficacy of systemic isotretinoin was superior to systemic minocycline and tetracycline and comparable to systemic minocycline given in combination with topical azelaic acid.

3. There is insufficient and conflicting evidence regarding the dose and cumulative dose of oral isotretinoin. Though majority of the trials have shown that higher doses are associated with better response, it also leads to less favourable safety/tolerability profile. The recommendations based on expert opinion and not on existing published trials on isotretinoin are:

   a. The recommended dose of oral isotretinoin for severe papulo-pustular and moderate nodular acne is 0.3–0.5 mg/kg body weight.

   b. The recommended dose of oral isotretinoin for conglobate acne is ≥ 0.5 mg/kg.

   c. The duration of the therapy with oral isotretinoin should be at least 6 months.

   d. The duration of treatment can be prolonged in case of insufficient response.

4. Consideration on isotretinoin and the risk of depression: Marqueling et al reported the rate of depression amongst isotretinoin users to range from 1% to 11% across trials, which was similar to those seen in oral antibiotic control groups (Marqueling & Zane LT, 2007). There is no statistically significant increase in the diagnosis of depression or depressive symptoms with the use of oral isotretinoin and no causative association between the two could be established. There is no correlation between use of isotretinoin and suicidal behaviour. However, patients should be informed regarding the possible risk of depression and suicidal behaviour with oral isotretinoin and history of depression in a patient should be taken for any patient before initiation of treatment and during treatment with isotretinoin.

5. There is still no conclusive evidence regarding the use of intense pulsed light, laser and photodynamic therapy in the treatment of conglobate acne.

6. There is scarcity of data regarding the safety and tolerability profile of different agents used for treating conglobate acne. Almost all the patients experience chelitis and xerosis with oral isotretinoin, while gastrointestinal side effects are commonly seen with oral antibiotics.

MAINTENANCE THERAPY IN ACNE

Topical retinoids are preferred for the maintenance therapy for the following reasons:

a. Retinoids prevent microcomedone formation and hence prevent development of new lesions

b. Their comedolytic action results in resolution of existing lesions; and

c. No development of bacterial resistance during long-term treatment.

Amongst the retinoids, *adapalene* is most widely used as maintenance therapy in various trials. Longer duration of therapy is likely to be successful as maintenance therapy. Due to its efficacy and favourable safety profile, topical *azelaic* acid can also serve as an alternate to topical retinoids for maintenance therapy (Graupe, 1996).

REFERENCES

1. Dominguez J, Hojyo MT, Celayo JL, Dominguez-Soto L, Teixeira F (1998). "Topical isotretinoin vs. topical retinoic acid in the treatment of acne vulgaris," Int J Dermatol 37:54–55.

2. Ellis CN, Leyden J, Katz HI et al (2001). "Therapeutic studies with a new combination benzoyl peroxide ? clindamycin topical gel in acne vulgaris," Cutis 67:13–20.

3. Garner SE, Eady EA, Popescu C, Newton J, Li WA (2003). "Minocycline for acne vulgaris: efficacy and safety. Cochrane Database Syst Rev(Online)," 1:CD002086.

4. Gollnick HP, Draelos Z, Glenn MJ et al (2009). "Adapalene-benzoyl peroxide, a unique fixed-dose combination topical gel for the treatment of acne vulgaris: a transatlantic, randomized, double-blind, controlled study in 1670 patients," Br J Dermatol 161: 1180–1189.

5. Gollnick HP, Graupe K, Zaumseil RP (2001). "Comparison of combined azelaic acid cream plus oral minocycline with oral isotretinoin in severe acne," Eur J Dermatol 11:538–544.

6. Graupe K, Cunliffe WJ, Gollnick HP, Zaumseil RP (1996). "Efficacy and safety of topical azelaic acid (20 percent cream): an overview of results from European clinical trials and experimental reports," Cutis 57:20–35.

7. Ioannides D, Rigopoulos D, Katsambas A (2002). "Topical adapalene gel 0.1% vs. isotretinoin gel 0.05% in the treatment of acne vulgaris: a randomized open-label clinical trial," Br J Dermatol 147:523–527.

8. Katsambas A, Graupe K, Stratigos J (1989). "Clinical studies of 20% azelaic acid cream in the treatment of acne vulgaris. Comparison with vehicle and topical tretinoin," Acta Derm Venereol Suppl (Stockh) 143:35–39.

9. Kellett N, West F, Finlay AY (2006). "Conjoint analysis: a novel, rigorous tool for determining patient preferences for topical antibiotic treatment for acne. A randomised controlled trial," Br J Dermatol 154:524–532.

10. Korkut C, Piskin S (2005). "Benzoyl peroxide, adapalene, and their combination in the treatment of acne vulgaris," J Dermatol 32: 169–173.

11. Layton AM (2001). "Optimal management of acne to prevent scarring and psychological sequelae," Am J Clin Dermatol 2:135–141.

12. Marqueling AL, Zane LT (2007). "Depression and suicidal behavior in acne patients treated with isotretinoin: a systematic review," Semin Cutan Med Surg 26:210–220.

13. Nast A, Dreno B, Bettoli V, Deditz K, Erdmann R, Finlay AY et al (2012). "European Evidence-based (S3) Guidelines for Treatment of Acne," J Eur Acad Dermatol Venereol 26 (Suppl. 1):1–29.

14. Nyirady J, Grossman RM, Nighland M et al (2001). "A comparative trial of two retinoids commonly used in the treatment of acne vulgaris," J Dermatolog Treat 12:149–157.

15. Rubinow DR, Peck GL, Squillace KM, Gantt GG (1987). "Reduced anxiety and depression in cystic acne patients after successful treatment with oral isotretinoin," J Am Acad Dermatol 17:25–32.

16. Smith K, Leyden JJ (2005). "Safety of doxycycline and minocycline: a systematic review," Clin Ther 27:1329–1342.

17. Zouboulis CC, Fischer TC, Wohlrab J, Barnard J, Alio AB (2009). "Study of the efficacy, tolerability, and safety of 2 fixed-dose combination gels in the management of acne vulgaris," Cutis 84: 223–229.

II. ACNE IN CHILDREN

INTRODUCTION

Acne vulgaris is a chronic disease that is virtually universal in adolescence and is the most common skin disease treated by physicians (Pochi PE, 1990). It is predominantly a dermatological problem in adolescents, but neonates, infants, and young children may also be affected (Jansen T *et al*, 1997). Appearance of acne in a young child may be a cause of concern for the parents. It may also be a sign of an underlying disorder. Although often dismissed as trivial, acne may lead to psychosocial morbidity, decreased quality of life and permanent scarring.

An understanding of acne pathogenesis helps the practitioner to conceptualize and formulate the therapeutic plan. Four interrelated processes, including hyperkeratinization, androgen stimulation, bacterial infection (*Propionibacterium acnes*), and inflammation are involved in this multifactorial disease. Certain exacerbating factors include stress, mechanical factors such as occlusion from sportsgear, topically applied preparations, especially pomades, greasy ointments, and cosmetics, and medications including corticosteroids, lithium, isoniazid, and hydantoin (Rothman KF, 1997). The role of diet in the pathogenesis of acne vulgaris remains controversial, and controlled studies have refuted the value of dietary restrictions (Thiboutot DM *et al*, 2002). Recently, the association between skim milk consumption and development of acne has been explored, with some studies suggesting a positive association, possibly related to a combination of exogenous hormones and growth factors, and stimulation of endogenous hormones (Adebamowo CA *et al*, 2008).

CLINICAL FEATURES

Categorization of paediatric acne: Both age and form of presentation are relevant to the diagnosis of pediatric acne. It can be classified into neonatal acne, infantile acne, midchildhood acne and prepubertal acne depending on the age of onset. The relevant age categories are presented in Table 5.4.

Table 5.4 *Paediatric acne categorized by age (Eichenfield et al, 2013)*	
Acne Type	*Age of Onset*
Neonatal	Birth to <6 weeks
Infantile	6 weeks to <1 year
Mid-childhood	1 year to 7 years
Pre-adolescent	>7 years to <12 years or menarche in girls
Adolescent	>12 years to < 19 years or after menarche in girls

Presenting History

The first step in patient evaluation is to gather a medical history (Box 1).

BOX 1. Important points in history

- Duration (early or late onset acne may indicate a hormonal abnormality)
- *Aggravating factors*:
  - Greasy applications/cosmetics (cosmetics containing lanolin or oil)
  - Any topical or systemic medication (topical or oral corticosteroids, isoniazid, hydantoin, or rifampin)
  - Recreational/Occupational activities (pressure applied by headband, tight occlusive garments, sports gear, e.g. helmets, chin straps, shoulder pads)
  - Any medical problem (hirsutism, atopics with dry skin may not tolerate acne medications)
  - Menstrual history in females (premenstrual flares common, oligo-menorrhea with hirsutism points towards hyperandrogenism)
- *Treatment history*:
  - Previous treatment with response (compliance, intolerance, adherence)

It is also important to know whether the patient is sexually active, or pregnant, in case the patient requires treatment with isotretinoin, though this does not apply to children. It is equally important to know, whether the patient is using any hormonal contraceptives as she may require additional contraceptive method if oral antibiotics are being used to treat acne.

Clinical Examination

Acne presents with a combination of the various lesion types as described in Table 5.5. At a minimum, the physical examination includes face, chest, back and upper arms. Examination of other systems will be dictated by history. To facilitate later comparison, an approximation of the number, and types of lesions along with scarring should be recorded for each geographic region. Acne can be categorized as predominately comedonal, inflammatory, and/or mixed. Presence or absence of scarring, post-inflammatory hyperpigmentation, or erythema should be assessed. Severity of acne may be broadly categorized as mild (comedones ± few papules/pustules), moderate (papules/pustules ± few nodules), or severe (nodular/conglobate). Photographic methods have been employed to assess disease activity and are preferred by some clinicians.

Table 5.5 *Important points in examination in acne*

Morphology	Sites of involvement	Other clinical signs
Open comedone (Blackheads)	Face	Hirsutism*
Closed comedone (Whiteheads)	Chest	Acanthosis nigricans*
Papule	Back	Female or male
Pustule	Upper arms	pattern alopecia*
Cyst		Truncal obesity
Nodule		Enlarged clitoris/
Dyspigmentation (usually		penis (signs of
hyperpigmentation)		precocious puberty)
Scarring (sometimes keloidal)*		

*not seen in children

NEONATAL ACNE (ACNE NEONATORUM)

Up to 20% of newborns can be affected by this condition in first few weeks of life (Marcoux D et al, 1998; Smolinski KN et al, 2004); males are affected more often than females (4–5:1). Neonatal acne may actually be a term used for a heterogeneous set of conditions presenting with papules and pustules, as well as true early acne presenting with comedones.

In this condition, erythematous papules or pustules appear mainly over the cheeks, chin, eyelids, and neck, but rarely upper chest, scalp and back may be involved. Usually, comedones are not seen (Cantatore Francis JL *et al 2006*, Niamba P *et al, 1998*) but early onset androgen driven acne can present with comedones. Neonatal acne may be hormonally mediated because newborns with neonatal acne present transient increase in circulating androgens. Meanwhile in the neonatal period, sebaceous glands are hyperplastic and increased androgenic activity of the glands may be responsible for neonatal acne development.

A neonatal pustular eruption termed 'neonatal cephalic pustulosis' presents in a similar fashion to neonatal acne. The condition is thought to occur due to the poral or follicular colonization by *Malassezia sympodialis* and *Malassezia globosa* (Niamba P *et al,* 1998; Bernier V *et al,* 2002; Bergman JN *et al,* 2002).The absence of comedones, the absence of follicular distribution, and monomorphic appearance of lesions distinguish it from neonatal acne. The disorder resolves spontaneously and treatment with topical ketoconazole or miconazole twice daily for 1–2 weeks is effective (Krowchuk DP *et al,* 2011).

INFANTILE ACNE (ACNE INFANTUM)

Infantile acne is a rare condition affecting children from 6 weeks to 1 year; however, some authors consider it to appear from the age of 6 months up to 16 months (Barnes CJ et al, 2005; Cunliffe WJ et al, 2001). It is more common in boys. Lesions of Infantile acne include closed and open comedones, papules, and pustules occasionally cysts and scar formation. Lesions generally resolve itself by 2 years of age. Infants with infantile acne are more prone to develop severe acne in their adolescence (Chew EW et al, 1990). Exact pathogenesis of infantile acne is still not known but it is thought to occur due to high level of production of dehydroepiandrosterone (DHEA) by fetal adrenal glands and this additional androgen production in boys further stimulates the sebaceous glands. High level of DHEA stimulates sebaceous gland up to 1year of age then it disappears and reappears at adrenarche (Jansen T et al, 1997; Lucky AW, 1998). Severe, persistent, or therapy- resistant infantile acne may be a sign of hyperandrogenism.

MID-CHILDHOOD ACNE

Acne in age group of 1–7 years is called mid-childhood acne. The appearance of acne in this age is *rare* and almost always points toward hyperandrogenism (Lucky AW, 1995). This is as there is virtually no adrenal or gonadal source of androgen in this developmental period. Its occurrence is rare because the production of androgen by fetal adrenal gland is maximum up to 1 year of age and then it stops, but recurs at adrenarche. The morphology of acne during this period includes open and closed comedones, inflammatory papules, pustules, cysts, and nodules. Distribution is primarily on the face and less often on the chest and back.

Thus in this age group the possibility of adrenal tumours, congenital adrenal hyperplasia, Cushing syndrome, gonadal or ovarian tumours, polycystic ovarian disease (PCOD), premature adrenarche, and true precocious puberty should be considered.

PREPUBERTAL ACNE (PRE-ADOLESCENT ACNE)

Prepubertal acne is the appearance of acne before true puberty, that is due to maturation of ovary and testis. Lesions of prepubertal acne mainly consist of comedones, with or without inflammatory lesions. Central area of the face (midforehead, nose, and chin, the "T-zone") is mainly affected as shown in Fig. 5.1, (Herane MI et al, 2003). Inflammatory papules and pustules usually present later and are relatively fewer in number. Presence of open comedones in the ear, (Fig. 5.2), which is often mistaken by parents for poor hygiene/dirt and scrubbed excessively. There may be significant progression in a

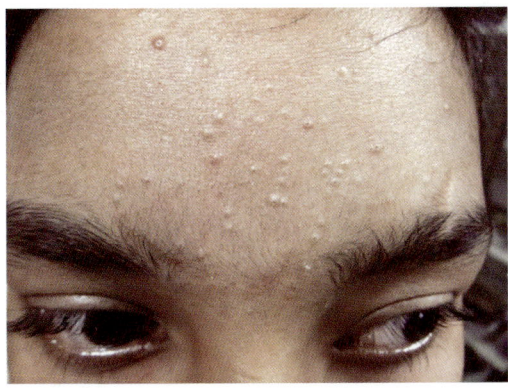

Fig. 5.1: Mild acne involving central area of the face

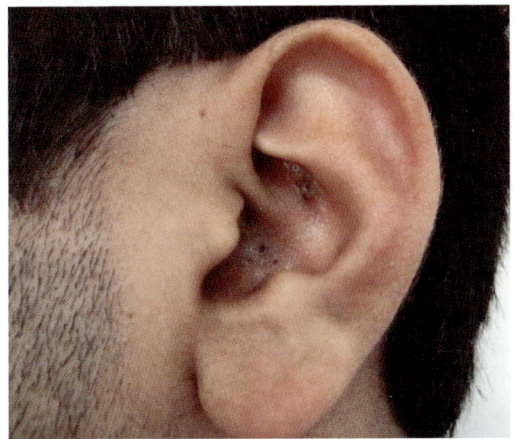

Fig. 5.2: The presence of open comedones in the ear, is a early sign of pediatric acne

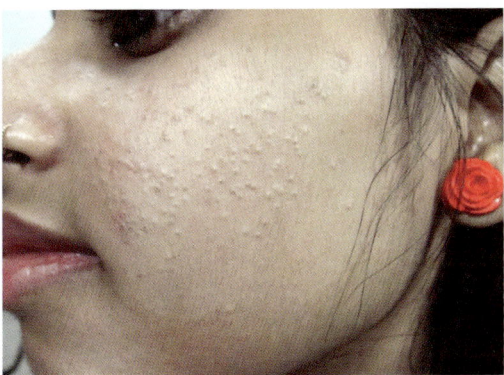

Fig. 5.3: Diffuse involvement of the face revealing comedonal acne

subgroup of these individuals from noninflammatory comedonal acne to severe, inflammatory disease with scarring (Fig. 5.3).

Acne can be the first sign of pubertal maturation in girls and may present before pubic hair and areolar development (Lucky AW *et al*, 1994). Age of adrenarche is 6–7 years in females and 7–8 years in males. During adrenarche, there is an increase in secretion of DHEA and dehydroepiandrosterone sulphate (DHEAS) by adrenal glands leading to activation of sebaceous gland. At this age, there is a little androgen production by the gonads and their maturation takes place 3–4 years after the adrenarche. Excess androgen production by ovary at this age can be due to benign or malignant tumour or more commonly due to PCOD.

ACNE VARIANTS

Acne excoriée: This form of acne is seen most commonly in adolescent females (*Bach M et al*). Patients manifest with crusting, scarring, and linear excoriations caused by scratching or picking their real or imagined acne lesions. The trauma can prolong the course of disease, and worsen inflammation and the scarring. It is best managed with emotional support and antibiotic therapy to prevent or treat secondary bacterial infection.

Periorificial dermatitis: In the pediatric age group, periorificial dermatitis occurs equally in boys and girls. Patients present with erythematous discrete papules and papulo-pustules in perioral, nasolabial and periocular locations. Its etiology is unknown, but it has been thought to represent a peculiar response to contact with topical fluorinated corticosteroids. In children, granulomatous form of periorificial dermatitis is seen where histopathology reveals upper dermal and perifollicular granulomas admixed with lymphocytes. It is generally self-limited. Treatment options of this condition include topical antibiotics (metronidazole, erythromycin) and, in more severe cases, oral erythromycin or tetracyclines (in patients >8 years).

Disorders associated with acne: Acne is an associated clinical manifestation in a number of pediatric disorders, namely Apert syndrome (acrocephalosyndactyly), SAPHO syndrome (synovitis, acne, pustulosis, hyperostosis, osteitis), and PAPA syndrome (sterile pyogenic arthritis, pyoderma gangranosum and acne).

INVESTIGATIONS

All patients of pediatric acne need not to be investigated. It has to be an individualized approach depending upon the age of presentation,

Table 5.6 *Approach in pediatric acne*		
Type of acne	*Indications of investigations*	*Investigations*
Neonatal and infantile acne	• Severe and persistent cases • Weight and height—if abnormal • Signs of precocious puberty (enlarged clitoris/ penis)	• Serum testosterone levels (free and total) • Serum dehydro-epiandrosterone sulphate level (DHEAS) • Serum luteinizing hormone (LH) • Serum follicle stimulating hormone (FSH)
Mid-childhood acne	• All cases (if onset is in this age) • Height and weight—if abnormal • Bone age—if abnormal • Signs of precocious puberty (enlarged clitoris/penis)	• Serum FSH • Serum LH • Serum testosterone (free and total) • Serum prolactin • Serum cortisol • Serum 17 α-hydroxy-progesterone
Prepubertal acne	• Recalcitrant acne • Menstrual irregularity • Hirsutism • Female or male pattern alopecia • Infertility • Acanthosis nigricans • Truncal obesity	• Ultrasonography of the pelvis • Serum testosterone (free and total) • Serum DHEAS • Serum LH • Serum FSH

severity, course, and additional signs and symptoms of any underlying disorder as dictated by history (Table 5.6).

DIAGNOSIS

The differential diagnosis of acne is presented in Table 5.7. Age of onset, lesion morphology, presence of comedones, and site of lesions are helpful to narrow down the options.

Treatment

Course of neonatal acne is benign and does not require any treatment except assurance to parents. Lesions resolve spontaneously without scarring.

Table 5.7 *Differential diagnosis of acne in pediatric and adolescent patients*

- Transient neonatal pustular melanosis ⎫
- Erythema toxicum neonatorum   ⎬ for neonatal acne
- Papulopustular eruption of hyper-IgE syndrome ⎭
- Acne venenata or pomade acne (from the use of topical or oil-based products)
- Bilateral nevus comedonicus
- Chlorinated aromatic hydrocarbons (chloracne)
- Corticosteroids (topical, inhaled, and oral)
- Demodex folliculitis
- Gram-negative folliculitis
- Malassezia (pityrosporum) folliculitis
- Papular sarcoidosis
- Facial angiofibromas (tuberous sclerosis)
- Flat warts
- Infections (bacterial, viral and fungal)
- Keratosis pilaris
- Medication-induced (anabolic steroids, dactinomycin, gold, isoniazid, lithium, phenytoin, and progestins)
- Milia
- Miliaria
- Molluscum contagiosum
- Periorificial dermatitis
- Rosacea
- Pseudofolliculitis barbae
- Tinea faciei
- Syringoma
- Sebaceous hyperplasia

Mild comedonal acne can be treated with topical tretinoins, and mild inflammatory disease is treated with 2.5% benzoyl peroxide or a topical antibiotic (1% clindamycin). More significant involvement may require treatment with oral antibiotics, usually erythromycin. However, in view of increasing resistance to erythromycin, other antibiotics such as azithromycin, and cephalexin can be used.

For infantile, mid-childhood, and pre-pubertal acne, therapeutic approach is same as that for acne in other age groups (Cantatore Francis JL *et al*, 2006 Antoniou C *et al*, 2009). An attempt should be made to

BOX 2. Key elements of patient education

No dietary restrictions are required for acne.

Frequent washing of face is not required.

Avoid picking of the acne lesions as it may cause scarring.

Pre-menstrual flare-ups can be seen in girls.

Greasy applications on face should be avoided.

Any mild soap can be used to wash the affected area.

Cosmetics, sunscreens, and moisturizers, especially those containing oils, may worsen acne. Noncomedogenic or gel-based cosmetics should be used.

Psychological stress may worsen acne.

Environmental factors like contact with greasy chemicals or excessive sweating may exacerbate acne.

address and dispel common myths and provide information about the behaviours and factors that may worsen acne.

The common topical and oral medications used for treating acne are summarised in Tables 5.8 and 5.9 respectively. Monotherapy should be avoided as this can lead to the development of resistance. Therefore, it is advisable to use topical antibiotics along with benzoyl peroxide or tretinoin (Paller AS *et al*, 2011). The treatment algorithms based on the acne severity are outlined in Table 5.10.

Systemic acne treatment, such as antibiotics, isotretinoin, and occasionally hormonal therapy, antiandrogens, can be added to the patient's regimen for more severe acne. For children of ages eight and above, after their dental enamel has been laid down, drugs of the tetracycline family (tetracycline, doxycycline, or minocycline) are safe options. If the patient has a tetracycline allergy, other options include erythromycin, clindamycin, trimethoprim-sulfamethoxazole, cephalexin, or amoxicillin. Similar to treatment of adolescent and adult acne, many practitioners will initiate treatment of moderate to severe acne in this age group with oral antibiotics, in combination with topical benzoyl peroxide and topical retinoids. Hormonal therapy, including estrogen-containing oral contraceptives, is not indicated in girls prior to menarche but can be a very useful adjuvant when more conventional treatment fails. For oral medication, it is also important to determine whether the patient is able to swallow pills; otherwise, liquid preparations, crushed tablets, or sprinkling of capsule contents on food are alternatives to be considered.

Intralesional injections of triamcinolone acetonide in low concentration (2.5 mg/kg) can be given for nodules and cysts (Cantatore Francis JL *et al*, 2006).

Table 5.8 Common topical medications used for acne

	Drug class/action	Common side effects	Contraindications
Tretinoin	1st Gen Retinoid, comedolytic	Xerosis, scaling, erythema, burning, contact dermatitis	Allergy
Adapalene	3rd Gen Retinoid, comedolytic	Xerosis, scaling, burning, erythema, photosensitivity	Allergy
Tazarotene	3rd Gen Retinoid, comedolytic contact dermatitis	Xerosis, scaling, erythema, burning,	Pregnancy
Clindamycin	Lincosamide antibiotic	Xerosis, erythema, burning	Allergy
Benzoyl peroxide	Oxidising agent, antibacterial and comedolytic	Xerosis, erythema, may bleach clothing	Allergy
Azelaic acid	Antibacterial, and anti-comedonal	Pruritus, burning, stinging, tingling, erythema	Allergy
Dapsone	Sulfone, anti-bacterial	Xerosis, erythema, contact dermatitis deficiency	Allergy Caution with G6PD

Table 5.9 Common oral medications used for acne

	Drug class	Common side effects	Contraindications
Doxycycline	Antibiotic	Photosensitivity, tooth discoloration, esophagitis, pseudotumour cerebri	Age <8 years old, pregnancy, allergy
Minocycline	Antibiotic	Hyperpigmentation, tooth discoloration, lupus-like syndrome, connective tissue disease, pseudo-tumour cerebri	Age <8 years old, pregnancy, allergy
Azithromycin	Antibiotic	Hepatotoxicity	Allergy, QT prolonga-tion, torsades de pointes
Erythromycin	Antibiotic	Gastrointestinal disturbances	Allergy

(contd.)

Table 5.9 *Common oral medications used for acne (contd.)*			
	Drug class	Common side effects	Contraindications
Trimethoprim/ sulfamethoxazole	Antibiotic	Stevens-Johnson syndrome, hepatic necrosis, aplastic anaemia, photosensitivity, hepatotoxicity, myelo-suppression	Allergy, hepatic impairment, G6PD deficiency, folate deficiency
Cephalexin	Antibiotic	Stevens-Johnson syndrome, neutropenia, thrombocyto-penia	Allergy
Isotretinoin	1st gen retinoid	Xerosis, cheilitis, photosensi-tivity, alopecia, skeletal hyperostosis, hypertrigly-ceridaemia, fatigue/ malaise, reversible mood changes, elevation of liver enzymes, inflammatory bowel disease, depression	Pregnancy, breast-feeding, allergy

Table 5.10 *Treatment algorithms (Eichenfield et al)*			
	Mild acne	Moderate acne	Severe acne
First-line treatment	• Benzoyl peroxide (BP) monotherapy • Retinoid monotherapy • BP + topical antibiotic • BP + retinoid • BP + topical antibiotic + retinoid	• BP + retinoid • BP + topical antibiotic + retinoid	• BP + oral anti-biotic + retinoid +/− topical antibiotic
Inadequate response	• Add BP or retinoid • Change retinoid concen-tration, type, or formulation • Change topical combina-tion therapy	• Change retinoid concentration, type, or formulation • Change topical combination therapy • Add oral antibiotic • Consider oral contraceptives • Consider oral isotretinoin	• Consider oral isotretinoin • Consider oral contraceptives

Isotretinoin is a Food and Drug Administration (FDA) approved drug for treatment of nodulocystic acne only in children of 12 years or older (Barnes CJ et al, 2005; Brecher AR et al, 2003), but there are published reports suggesting successful role of isotretinoin in younger children. Dose of isotretinoin for infantile acne is not known but dose range of 0.2–2.0 mg/kg/day divided in two daily doses for 4–14 months in children up to 5 years of age can be used (Barnes CJ et al, 2005; Cunliffe WJ et al, 2001; Arbegast KD et al, 1991; Horne HL et al, 1997; Sarazin F et al, 2004; Torrelo A et al, 2005). As isotretinoin is available in capsules, it is problematic to administer it in children. The problem can be overcome by opening the capsule in dim light and mixing the contents with soft food like cheese and butter (Torrelo A et al, 2005). The capsule should never be opened in light as isotretinoin is very labile to light and heat. Another way of administration of the capsule is to freeze it till it becomes solid and then cut the capsule up to desired dose and mix it with palatable food. Liver function tests, serum lipid profile, complete blood count and skeletal growth should be monitored regularly while patient is on isotretinoin. Premature epiphyseal closure is unlikely to occur at such low doses used in the treatment of acne. Hormonal therapy is considered when etiology of acne is CAH or polycystic ovary syndrome. Oral contraceptives or antiandrogen can be prescribed in case of PCOD. For CAH, low doses of oral corticosteroids are given (Lucky AW et al, 1994). If benign or malignant tumour of the ovary is the underlying cause of acne, then gynaecological referral is recommended.

CONCLUSION

The manifestations of acne vary according to age. Neonatal acne is self-limiting and rarely needs any treatment. Infantile acne can be a predictor of more severe acne in adolescence. In the treatment of childhood acne, contraindication of oral tetracyclines should be considered. Use of oral isotretinoin has proven to be successful in infantile and midchildhood acne but currently it is FDA approved only for children above 12 years of age. Further studies are needed to prove its safety in children in doses used for adult acne. Severe acne in children of any age warrants careful evaluation to rule out endocrinal abnormalities.

REFERENCES

1. Adebamowo CA, Spiegelman D, Berkey CS, et al. Milk consumption and acne in teenaged boys. J Am Acad Dermatol.2008; 58:787–93.

2. Antoniou C, Dessinioti C, Stratigos AJ, Katsambas AD. Clinical and therapeutic approach to childhood acne: An update. *Pediatr Dermatol* 2009; 26:373–80.

3. Arbegast KD, Braddock SW, Lamberty LF, Sawka AR. Treatment of infantile cystic acne with oral isotretinoin: A case report. *Pediatr Dermatol* 1991; 8:16–68.

4. Bach M, Bach D. Psychiatric and psychometric issues in acne excoriée. *Psychother psychosom.* 1993; 60:207–10.

5. Barnes CJ, Eichenfield LF, Lee J, Cunningham BB. A practical approach for the use of oral isotretinoin for infantile acne. *Pediatr Dermatol* 2005; 22: 166–9.

6. Bergman JN, Eichenfield LF. Neonatal acne and cephalic pustulosis: Is *Malassezia* the whole story? *Arch Dermatol* 2002; 138:255–7.

7. Bernier V, Weill FX, Hirigoyen V, Elleau C, Feyler A, Labrèze C, *et al.* Skin colonization by *Malassezia* species in neonates: A prospective study and relationship with neonatal cephalic pustulosis. *Arch Dermatol* 2002; 138:215–8.

8. Brecher AR, Orlow SJ. Oral retinoid therapy for dermatologic conditions in children and adolescents. *J Am Acad Dermatol* 2003;49:171–82.

9. Cantatore Francis JL, Glick SA. Childhood acne: Evaluation and management. *Dermatol Ther* 2006; 19:202–9.

10. Chew EW, Bingham A, Burrows D. Incidence of acne vulgaris in patients with infantile acne. *Clin Exp Dermatol* 1990; 15:376–7.

11. Cunliffe WJ, Baron SE, Coulson IH. A clinical and therapeutic study of 29 patients with infantile acne. *Br J Dermatol* 2001; 145:463–6.

12. Eichenfield LF, Krakowski AC, Piggott C, *et al.* Evidence-based recommendations for the diagnosis and treatment of pediatric acne. *Pediatrics.* 2013; 131 Suppl 3:S163–86.

13. Herane MI, Ando I. Acne in infancy and acne genetics. *Dermatology* 2003; 206:24–8.

14. Horne HL, Carmichael AJ. Juvenile nodulocystic acne responding to systemic isotretinoin. *Br J Dermatol* 1997; 136:796–7.

15. Jain AK, Morgaonkar M. Acne in childhood: Clinical presentation, evaluation and treatment *Indian J Pediatr Dermatol* 2015; 16:1–4.

16. Jansen T, Burgdorf WH, Plewig G. Pathogenesis and treatment of acne in childhood. *Pediatr Dermatol* 1997; 14:172–1.

17. Krowchuk DP, Gelmetti C, Lucky AW. Acne In: Schachner LA, Hansen RC, editors. *Pediatric Dermatology.* 4th ed. Philadelphia: Elsevier; 2011:827–50.

18. Lucky AW. A review of infantile and pediatric acne. *Dermatology* 1998; 196:95–7.

19. Lucky AW. Hormonal correlates of acne and hirsutism. *Am J Med* 1995; 98:89–94.

20. Lucky AW, Biro FM, Huster GA, Leach AD, Morrison JA, Ratterman J. Acne vulgaris in premenarchal girls. An early sign of puberty associated with rising levels of dehydroepiandrosterone. *Arch Dermatol* 1994; 130:308–14.

21. Marcoux D, McCuaig CC, Powell J. Prepubertal acne: Clinical presentation, evaluation, and treatment. *J Cutan Med Surg* 1998;2 Suppl 3:2–6.

22. Niamba P, Weill FX, Sarlangue J, Labrèze C, Couprie B, Taïeh A. Is common neonatal cephalic pustulosis (neonatal acne) triggered by *Malassezia sympodialis? Arch Dermatol* 1998; 134: 995–8.

23. Paller AS, Mancini AJ, editors. Disorders of the sebaceous and sweat glands. In: *Hurwitz Clinical Pediatric Dermatology.* 4th ed. Philadelphia: WB Saunders; 2011:167–83.

24. Pochi PE: The pathogenesis and treatment of acne. *Annu Rev Med.* 1990; 41:187–98.

25. Rapelanoro R, Mortureux P, Couprie B, Maleville J, Taïeb A. Neonatal *Malassezia furfur* pustulosis. *Arch Dermatol* 1996; 132:190–3.

26. Rothman KF: Acne update. *Dermatol Ther.* 1997; 2:98–110.

27. Sarazin F, Dompmartin A, Nivot S, Letessier D, Leroy D. Treatment of an infantile acne with oral isotretinoin. *Eur J Dermatol* 2004; 14:71–2.

28. Smolinski KN, Yan AC. Acne update: 2004. *Curr Opin Pediatr* 2004; 16:385–91.

29. Thiboutot DM, Strauss JS. Diet and acne revisited. *Arch Dermatol.* 2002; 138:1591–2.

30. Torrelo A, Pastor MA, Zambrano A. Severe acne infantum successfully treated with isotretinoin. *Pediatr Dermatol* 2005; 22:357–9.

III. TREATMENT GUIDELINES IN ADULT WOMEN

This chapter gives an overview of guidelines of acne in women as this topic has been addressed under the heading of hormonal and post-adolescent acne.

In adult females a substantial focus is on the role of androgens in acne. Though some studies have shown high levels of androgens, others have opined that even if they are within normal limits, the serum level of circulating androgens is significantly increased in women with acne compared with women without acne (Cibula D, 2000; Thiboutot D, 1999). The severity of acne may also be related to the sexual maturity of males and females, which may be associated to an increase in sensitivity of the sebaceous gland to androgens (Beylot C, 1998; Lucky AW, 1997). Women with severe seborrhea, clinically apparent androgenic alopecia, seborrhea/acne/hirsutism/alopecia (SAHA) syndrome, late-onset acne (acne tarda), and proven ovarian or adrenal hyperandrogenism may benefit from hormonal therapy (Gollnick H, 2003).

Which Patients are Ideal Candidates for Hormonal Investigations?

i. Acne that is resistant to conventional therapy.

ii. A sudden onset of severe acne.

iii. Acne associated with clinical signs of virilization, irregular menses, or signs of hyperandrogenism (SAHA syndrome).

iv. Relapsing acne lesions shortly after isotretinoin therapy (Gollnick H, 2003).

v. Adult women and sexually active teens with premenstrual acne flares (Thiboutot DM, 2001).

vi. Combined oral contraceptive (OC) therapy can also be used as first-line therapy for hirsutism and acne in women with PCOS (Gollnick H, 2003).

vii. Women with late onset of acne (acne tarda) or persistant acne.

viii. Prominance of acne on lower face and neck.

The most common endocrinopathies associated with acne include polycystic ovary syndrome (PCOS), late-onset adrenal hyperplasia (LOAH), or a virilizing tumour. Additionally, hormonal therapy can be effective in women with normal androgen levels (Katsambas AD, 2010).

CLINICAL SIGNS OF HORMONAL ABNORMALITIES

1. Acneiform lesions along the mandible and chin which often flare that correlate with their menstrual cycles (Olutunmbi Y, 2008). These

women usually do not have increased androgen levels above normal.

2. Signs of virilization (e.g. hirsutism).

3. Symptoms of androgen excess include menstrual irregularity, infertility, hirsutism, truncal obesity, polycystic ovaries detected on sonogram, recalcitrant acne, infrequent menses, female-pattern or male-pattern alopecia, deepening of voice, and cliteromegaly.

4. HAIR-AN syndrome: Hirsutism or irregular menstrual periods, acanthosis nigricans (e.g. HAIR-AN syndrome: hyperandrogenism, insulin resistance, and acanthosis nigricans) should warrant hormonal screening.

PCOS

PCOS was previously defined according to the proceedings of an expert conference sponsored by the National Institutes of Health (NIH) in 1990, which described the disorder as including hyperandrogenism or hyperandrogenemia (*or both*), oligo-ovulation, and exclusion of known disorders of androgen excess and anovulation. Another expert conference held in Rotterdam in 2003 defined PCOS, after the exclusion of related disorders, by the presence of *two* of the following three features: oligo-ovulation or anovulation, clinical or biochemical signs of hyperandrogenism (or both), and polycystic ovaries (Box 3).

In essence, the Rotterdam 2003 criteria expanded the NIH 1990 definition by creating four new phenotypes: Ovulatory women with

---

BOX 3. 1990 National Institutes of Health criteria and 2003 Rotterdam criteria for the diagnosis of polycystic ovary syndrome

National Institutes of Health criteria (requires all 3):
1. Chronic anovulation.
2. Clinical and/or biochemical signs of hyperandrogenism.
3. Exclusion of other causes of hyperandrogenism and anovulation, such as Cushing syndrome, congenital adrenal hyperplasia, and androgen-secreting tumours.

Rotterdam criteria (requires 2 out of 3):
1. Oligo- or anovulation.
2. Clinical and/or biochemical signs of hyperandrogenism.
3. Echogenic evidence of polycystic ovaries and exclusion of other causes of hyperandrogenism and anovulation, such as Cushing syndrome, congenital adrenal hyperplasia, and androgen-secreting tumours.

BOX 4. Polycystic ovary syndrome phenotypes based on the 2003 Rotterdam criteria

Phenotype	Prevalence	Clinical features
Severe PCOS	61%	Irregular menses, polycystic ovaries, hyperandrogenemia, and hyperinsulinemia
Hyperandrogenism and chronic anovulation	7%	Irregular menses, normal ovaries, hyperandrogenemia, and hyperinsulinemia
Ovulatory PCOS	16%	Normal menses, polycystic ovaries, hyperandrogenemia, and hyperinsulinemia
Mild PCOS	16%	Irregular menses, polycystic ovaries, mildly raised androgen levels, and normal insulin levels

polycystic ovaries plus hyperandrogenism and oligo-anovulatory women with polycystic ovaries but without hyperandrogenism (Box 4).

Importantly hyperandrogenism, is identified clinically as hirsutism (modified Ferriman-Gallway score FGS > 6), acne, seborrhea, and less commonly hair loss, while hyperandrogenemia is defined as a free testosterone serum level greater than 2.7 pg/ml and/or total testosterone greater than 80 ng/dl. In our patients, with adult women acne, acne itself is not a sign of hyperandrogenism. But as per the new criterion of PCOS, even in patients without marked hirsutism, PCOS is a possibility. Thus in essence clinically normal patients of acne with history of irregular menses should be investigated for PCOS.

HOW TO INVESTIGATE?

This has been detailed previously and a summary is given here:
1. Screening tests for hyperandrogenism should be obtained in the luteal phase of the menstrual cycle.
2. They include serum dehydroepiandrosterone (DHEAS), total testosterone, free testosterone, luteinizing hormone/follicle-stimulating hormone (LH/FSH) ratio (not necessary for diagnosis now though still helpful), prolactin, and 17-hydroxyprogesterone. We also use the levels of anti-Müllerian hormone (AMH) with a cut off 4 ng/ml being suggestive of PCOS.

Interpretation

1. Normal total testosterone and DHEAS levels are the commonest finding in patients with acne.

2. A raised AMH, high normal testosterone and low sex hormone binding globulin (SHBG) is seen in PCOS testosterone. LH:FSH has a little role in obese PCOS patients, thus its absence is not considered to be important in all cases of PCOS.

3. High levels of testosterone >150 to 200 ng/dL are seen in tumours.

4. Serum DHEAS >8000 ng/mL is highly suggestive of an adrenal tumour, while a value of 4000 to 8000 ng/mL may indicate congenital adrenal hyperplasia.

5. In women, transvaginal ultrasound accurately measures the follicle size and number. But since it should not be done in unmarried women, transabdominal ultrasound is done and it is more accurate in measuring the ovarian volume than follicle size and number. Hence importance should be given to ovarian volume in unmarried women in diagnosing PCOS. This is specially important in our cultural set up.

TREATMENT

A. Antiandrogens

Antiandrogens, or androgen receptor blockers, competitively inhibit the binding of dihydrotestosterone to its receptor and include cyproterone acetate (CPA), drospirenone, spironolactone, and flutamide (Faure M).

1. *Cyproterone acetate (CPA):* CPA (10 mg, 50 mg) is a progestational antiandrogen that inhibits binding of dihydrotestosterone to its receptor. It reduces the activity of 5α-reductase, preventing the transformation of testosterone to dihydrotestosterone. It also blocks ovarian function and decreases serum androgen levels by inhibiting production of FSH and LH. Treatment with CPA should begin on the first day of the menstrual cycle.

CPA at a dose of 50 to 100 mg daily (with or without EE 50 mg) has been shown to result in improvement in 75% to 90% of patients treated (van Wayjen RG). Since giving CPA alone causes menstrual irregularities, it is best combined with an OCP.

CPA is usually prescribed at doses between 2 and 100 mg daily and is often combined with ethinyl estradiol (EE) in the form of a oral contraceptive (OC) (Dronis 30/Diane 35) that is approved in Europe and India for the treatment of acne.

Reported side effects include menstrual abnormalities, breast tenderness and enlargement, nausea/vomiting, fluid retention, leg edema, headache, and melasma. Other side effects include fatigue, changes in body weight, liver dysfunction, and rarely, blood-clotting disorders.

2. *Spironolactone* is an androgen receptor blocker, 5α-reductase inhibitor, and aldosterone antagonist that has been used for the treatment of hirsutism and hypertension. The US Food and Drug

Administration has not formally approved use of spironolactone for the treatment of acne; however, it may be used for females who have failed other therapeutic interventions.

Dose: 50 to 100 mg twice daily, it exerts its effects by blocking androgen receptors and has been shown to reduce sebum production by 30% to 50% leading to decreased acne production (Goodfellow A, 1984; Akamatsu H, 1993). *Low doses* of 25 mg twice daily or 25 mg daily may be sufficient for women with sporadic outbreaks of inflammatory lesions or isolated cysts. *Maintenance* doses range from 25 to 50 mg daily. Additionally, use of spironolactone in combination with an OC pill containing 30 mg EE/3 mg drospirenone has been shown to be effective and well tolerated (Krunic A, 2008).

Spironolactone in low doses is generally well tolerated. However, use of spironolactone at higher doses or in females with cardiac or renal dysfunction may result in hyperkalemia. Other side effects include menstrual irregularity, breast tenderness, gynecomastia, headache, and fatigue. Spironolactone is contraindicated in women who are pregnant or at increased risk of breast cancer.

3. *Flutamide* is a nonsteroidal antiandrogen used for the management of prostatic hypertrophy, prostate cancer, and hirsutism. For the treatment of acne or hirsutism in females, it has been used at doses of 250 mg twice a day in combination with OCs. In a study comparing spironolactone and flutamide therapy in the treatment of acne, flutamide therapy was shown to have a greater effect at reducing total acne and seborrhea after three months. However, it is infrequently prescribed due to its hepatotoxicity.

B. Inhibitors of Ovarian Androgen Production

OCPs are the simplest and most effective agents for inhibiting ovarian androgen production. They are indicated in the following scenarios:

1. In women who desire oral contraception and those who are concurrently being treated with isotretinoin.
2. Women with premenstrual flare of acne, during treatment with isotretinoin, or when oral contraception is desired.
3. Women whose acne does not respond to other therapeutic interventions.
4. Women with polycystic ovary syndrome.
5. Women with clinical signs of hyperandrogenism.
6. Women with late-onset acne
7. Women with proven ovarian hyperandrogenism.

Principles of Use

The "trick" is not to use andogenic progesterones. Earlier generations of progestins used in OCs (e.g. estrane and gonane classes) have been reported to cross-react with androgen receptors resulting in androgenic effects and increased acne, specifically at higher doses than that which is present in newer OCs. Second-generation progestins such as ethynodiol diacetate, norethindrone, and levonorgestrel have the lowest androgenic activity. The third-generation progestins, including norgestimate, desogestrel, and gestodene, are more selective for the progesterone receptor and have the lowest androgenic activity since these agents are metabolized to levonorgestrel. Drospirenone, a progestin derived from spironolactone, has antiandrogenic and antimineralocorticoid activity and improves acne, hirsutism, and estrogen-related fluid retention associated with some OCs (Thorneycroft IH, 2002). It has no androgenic potential. It is my preferred OCP fixed drug combination (FDC).

The *mode of action* is, by (i) their ability to suppress ovarian production of androgens, which reduces serum androgen levels and sebum production, (ii) suppressing the secretion of pituitary gonadotropins, thereby reducing ovarian androgen production, or (iii) increasing liver synthesis of SHBH, resulting sex hormone binding globulin, resulting in the decrease of free serum testosterone.

The use of OCs (20 mg of EE/100 mg of levonorgestrel, 35 mg EE/norgestimate) has been shown to be effective and safe for the treatment of acne in women (Redmond GP, 1997). Reduction in inflammatory lesions by 30 to 60%, improvement of acne in 50% to 90% of patients, and noninflammatory facial acne lesions have been shown following six to nine months of use (Arowojolu AO, 2004). Additionally, OCs containing drospirenone have been shown to be superior to a triphasic OC containing EE/norgestimate in the treatment of acne and had comparable efficacy to Diane-35 (Thorneycroft H, 2004).

A list of common OCP in India are detailed in Box 5.

Estrogen /Drosperinone Use in OCP

The contraceptive pill has been a revolution of the last 40 years. Although reduction in the concentration of ethinyl estradiol (EE) has reduced the incidence of negative systemic side effects such as water retention, edema and swollen breasts, the **low estrogen dose** may be associated with *spotting and hypomenorrhea or amenorrhea* in the long term, as well as *dyspareunia* due to reduced vaginal trophism, which may induce women to suspend use of the drug.

The choice of *progesterone* therefore involves not only its effect on the endometrium in synergy with estrogen, but also possible residual androgenic activity which may have negative metabolic repercussions. Indeed, addition of a progesterone, especially androgen-derived, attenuates the positive metabolic effects of estrogen. Two new monophasic oral contraceptives were recently released. They contain

BOX 5. A list of common OCP in India

Brand Name	Composition	Androgenic Activity*
BANDHAN	Ethinylestradiol 0.03 mg, Levonorgestrel 0.15 mg	Levonorgestrel 1 mg = 8.3
MALA-D TAB	Ethinylestradiol 0.03 mg, Norgestrel 0.30 mg	Norgestrel 1 mg = 4.2
OVARAL-L TAB	Ethinylestradiol 0.03 mg, Levonorgestrel 0.15 mg	Levonorgestrel 1 mg = 8.3
FEMILON TAB	Ethinyloestradiol 0.02 mg, Desogestrel 0.15 mg	Desogestrel 1 mg = 3.4
NOVELON TAB	Ethinyloestradiol 0.03 mg, Desogesterel 0.15 mg	Desogestrel 1 mg = 3.4
DRONIS-20	Ethinyloestradiol 0.02 mg, Drospirenone 3 mg	Drospirenone 1 mg = 0
DRONIS-30/Yasmin	Ethinyloestradiol 0.03 mg, Drospirenone 3 mg	Drospirenone 1 mg = 0

*Relative to 1 mg of norethindrone

30 µg or 20 µg EE and a new progesterone, drospirenone, derived from spironolactone, which has antiandrogenic and antimineralocorticoid activity similar to endogenous progesterone.

Like progesterone, the drospirenone molecule is an aldosterone antagonist and has a natriuretic effect that opposes the sodium retention effect of EE. It may, therefore, help to prevent the water retention, weight gain and arterial hypertension often associated with oral contraceptive use. Recent comparative studies recorded weight loss that stabilized after 6 months of treatment with drospirenone/EE.

1. *Overweight women* may therefore benefit from the formulation with 20 µg EE, whereas the formulation with at least 30 µg EE should be more appropriate for *underweight women.*

2. In women with mild to moderate acne, with slight to moderate acne, the formulation with 30 µg EE has been found to be as effective as 2 mg cyproterone acetate combined with 35 µg EE (Diane-35).

3. *Menstrual cycle* characteristics, however, remain the main factor determining the choice of formulation. Randomised control studies comparing the new formulation with others containing second or third generation progesterones have found similar efficacy in cycle control and incidence of spotting.

Thus if a women has *normal* cycles *30 µg EE* is enough. In cases of *hypomenorrhea and/or amenorrhea* at least this dose of EE plus drospirenone may be used.

Women with *hypermenorrhea* run the risk of spotting if an inappropriate drug is chosen. A solution is to use *30 µg EE/ drospirenone* from day 5 of the cycle. To control so-called minor side-effects, the dose of EE must be appropriate.

4. In women with *premenstrual tension* a dose of at least *30 µg EE* associated with drospirenone reduces or even prevents symptoms.
5. In cases of *chronic headache or headache* as a side-effect of oral contraceptive use, a lower dose of estrogen is beneficial, and doses below 20 µg may be used. Although the progesterone component is not considered to affect headache, good results have been obtained with drospirenone, the anti-mineralocorticoid effects of which reduce blood pressure and improve symptoms.
6. Formulations with *20 µg EE* and drospirenone are particularly indicated in women with pre-existing *mastodynia, fibrocystic breast manifestations* or who develop mastodynia as a side-effect of oral contraceptive use. Since high plasma concentrations of androgens have been recorded in these women, a progesterone with antiandrogen and antiedema activity can be beneficial.
7. Finally, it is worth recalling that monophasic pills with low estrogen doses, such as the formulations mentioned above, ensure good mood control, reducing the depressive symptoms often associated with oral contraceptive use. In conclusion, formulations containing drospirenone are a valid alternative to conventional oral contraceptives for the personalisation of these drugs.

C. Blocking Adrenal Androgen Production

Low-dose glucocorticoids effectively suppresses the adrenal production of androgens and are indicated for use in patients (male or female) who have an elevated serum DHEAS, often associated with 11- or 21-hydroxylase deficiency.

In acute flares of acne or in severe acne, glucocorticoids may be used in low doses (prednisone 2.5 or 5 mg or dexamethasone 0.25 or 0.75 mg) daily or every other day to suppress adrenal androgen production. It should be noted that patients treated with dexamethasone are at particularly higher risk for adrenal suppression. During treatment, patients should be followed closely for signs of adrenal suppression with ACTH (cosyntropin) stimulation tests performed two to three months after initiation of therapy.

D. Gonadotropin-releasing Hormone Agonists

GnRH agonists inhibit ovarian androgen production by blocking the cyclic release of LH and FSH from the pituitary, leading to the suppression of ovarian steroidogenesis. GnRH agonists include agents such as nafarelin, leuprolide, and buserelin, which are only available as nasal sprays or injectables.

The use of GnRH agonists is limited by their expense and side effects, including ovarian estrogen suppression and the development of menopausal symptoms, headaches, and bone loss.

CONCLUSIONS

It must be remembered that hormonal therapy is not effective as a monotherapy. They take time to work and atleast 6 months of therapy should be given (Nast A, 2012). They should be combined with oral isotretinoin, oral antibiotics, topical retinoids, or benzoyl peroxide depending on the severity of acne. In case of PCOS , there are other therapies required and in essence the OCP has to be continued for atleast 6 months and sometimes longer to have an appreciable effect in hormonal acne.

REFERENCES

1. Akamatsu H, Zouboulis CC, Orfanos CE. Spironolactone directly inhibits proliferation of cultured human facial sebocytes and acts antagonistically to testosterone and 5 alpha dihydrotestosterone in vitro. J Invest Dermatol 1993; 100(5):660–662.

2. Arowojolu AO, Gallo MF, Grimes DA, et al. Combined oral contraceptive pills for treatment of acne. Cochrane Database Syst Rev 2004; (3):CD0044–25.

3. Beylot C, Doutre MS, Beylot Barry M. Oral contraceptives and cyproterone acetate in female acne treatment. Dermatology 1998; 196(1):148–152.

4. Cibula D, Hill M, Vohradnikova O, et al. The role of androgens in determining acne severity in adult women. Br J Dermatol 2000; 143(2):399–404.

5. Faure M, Drapier Faure E. [Hormonal treatments of acne]. Ann Dermatol Venereol 2003; 130(1 pt 2):142–147.

6. Gollnick H, Cunliffe W, Berson D, et al. Management of acne: A report from a Global Alliance to Improve Outcomes in Acne. J Am Acad Dermatol 2003; 49(1 suppl):S1–S37.

7. Goodfellow A, Alaghband Zadeh J, Carter G, et al. Oral spironolactone improves acne vulgaris and reduces sebum excretion. Br J Dermatol 1984; 111(2):209–214.

8. Katsambas AD, Dessinioti C. Hormonal therapy for acne: why not as first line therapy? Facts and controversies. Clin Dermatol 2010; 28(1):17–23.

9. Krunic A, Ciurea A, Scheman A. Efficacy and tolerance of acne treatment using both spironolactone and a combined contraceptive containing drospirenone. J Am Acad Dermatol 2008; 58(1):60–62.

10. Lucky AW, Henderson TA, Olson WH, et al. Effectiveness of norgestimate and ethinyl estradiol in treating moderate acne vulgaris. J Am Acad Dermatol 1997; 37(5 pt 1):746–754.

11. Nast A, Dreno B, Bettoli V, Deditz K, Erdmann R, Finlay AY et al (2012). "European Evidence-based (S3) Guidelines for Treatment of Acne," J Eur Acad Dermatol Venereol 26; (Suppl. 1):1–29.

12. Olutunmbi Y, Paley K, English JC III. Adolescent female acne: etiology and management. J Pediatr Adolesc Gynecol 2008; 21(4):171–176.

13. Redmond GP, Olson WH, Lippman JS, et al. Norgestimate and ethinyl estradiol in the treatment of acne vulgaris: a randomized, placebo controlled trial. Obstet Gynecol 1997; 89(4):615–622.

14. Thiboutot D, Gilliland K, Light J, et al. Androgen metabolism in sebaceous glands from subjects with and without acne. Arch Dermatol 1999; 135(9):1041–1045.

15. Thiboutot DM. Endocrinological evaluation and hormonal therapy for women with difficult acne. J Eur Acad Dermatol Venereol 2001; 15(suppl 3):57–61.

16. Thorneycroft H, Gollnick H, Schellschmidt I. Superiority of a combined contraceptive containing drospirenone to a triphasic preparation containing norgestimate in acne treatment. Cutis 2004; 74(2):123–130.

17. Thorneycroft IH. Evolution of progestins. Focus on the novel progestin drospirenone. J Reprod Med 2002; 47(11 suppl):975–980.

18. van Wayjen RG, van den Ende A. Experience in the long term treatment of patients with hirsutism and/or acne with cyproterone acetate containing preparations: Efficacy, metabolic and endocrine effects. Exp Clin Endocrinol Diabetes 1995; 103(4): 241–251.

6

Acne Variants and Scenarios

I. ACNE CONGLOBATA

INTRODUCTION

Reitmann, Spitzer and Lang separately described the morphology and histology of this condition initially. Acne conglobata is one of the severe forms of acne characterized by polyporous blackheads, burrowing abscesses and irregular scarring. The challenges posed by this variant is its chronicity, severity and difficulty in treatment.

What causes acne conglobata, is still unknown. Some causes that are implicated include anabolic/androgenic steroid use, androgen-producing tumours, and testosterone therapy [Melnik B, 2007]. Environmental factors have been implicated including exposure to halogenated hydrocarbons or ingestion of halogens. Chromosomal defects have been found in some patients with acne conglobata, namely an XXY karyotype in individuals.

Patients with acne conglobata are predominantly males, usually between ages of 18 and 30 with extensive acne characterized by severe nodular in ammation and scarring. If it is seen in females a possible cause is a hormonal dysfunction.

Clinical Features

This condition frequently starts de novo but may possibly develop from existing active papular or pustular acne. It is charactersied by numerous comedones, papules, pustules, nodules, abscesses, and draining sinus tracts involving mainly the chest, back, and buttocks (Fig. 6.1). A *hallmark* of this disease is the presence of grouped comedones, mainly on the posterior neck and upper trunk. The nodules gradually increase size and break down to discharge pus. When the

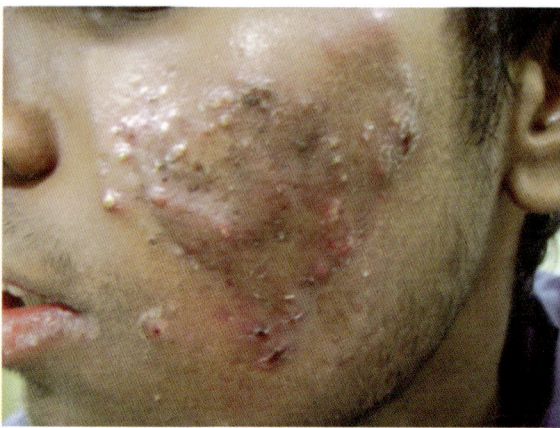

Fig. 6.1: A case of acne conglobata with edema, papules, pustules, nodules and cysts on the face

nodules break down, crusts may cover an indolent deep ulcer which tends to extend centrifugally with centred healing. Draining sinuses may be seen in the form of a persistent lesion of linear or angular shape with a discharge of pus or blood. Sinus tracts have multiple orifices, nodules and granulomatous inflammation. This condition persists for years, with no tendency to spontaneous resolution. Disfiguring scars, which are usually atrophic but occasionally keloidal, may accompany the progressive extension of the lesions and many cases remain active for 25 years or more (Fig. 6.2). Histologically, inflammatory infiltrate is present around follicles, which can often disrupt the normal dermal architecture.

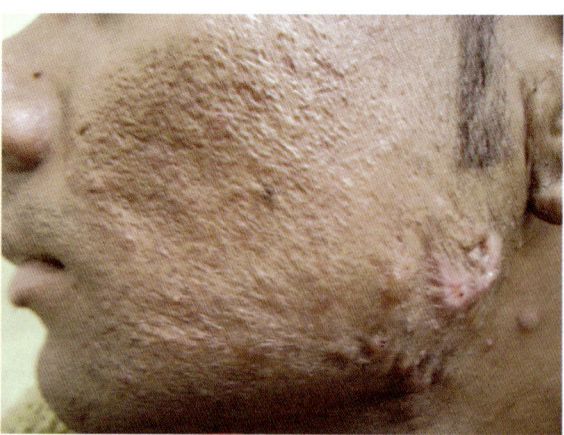

Fig. 6.2: Unfortunate sequelae of a case of acne conglobata with scarring. This dictates the urgency of aggressive treatment of such conditions

Acne conglobata (AC) resembles acne fulminans in causing widespread inflammatory nodules on the trunk. Acne conglobata produces polyporus comedones and noninflammatory cysts, while acne fulminans does not. Unlike acne conglobata, large nodules of acne fulminans tend to become painful ulcers with overhanging borders surrounding exudative necrotic plaques that become confluent. Also peripheral neutrophilia is not seen in acne conglobata

Acne conglobata may be associated with secondary obstruction and inflammation of the apocrine units of the axilla, breast and perineum producing hidradenitis suppurativa (*acne inversa*). Acne conglobata may occur in association with hidradenitis suppurativa as part of the follicular occlusion triad (acne conglobata, hidradenitis suppurativa, and dissecting cellulitis of the scalp) [Chicarilli ZN, 1987]. This is also known as the follicular occlusion tetrad, constituting acne conglobata, hidradenitis suppurativa, and dissecting cellulitis of the scalp, pilonidal sinus [Vasanth V, 2014].

Investigations

Acne conglobata is generally a clinical diagnosis. A good history and physical to rule out acne fulminans is indicated.

1. In women, the presence of acne conglobata may indicate the need for an endocrinologic work-up to include total and free testosterone, DHEAS, prolactin, LH and FSH (Fig. 6.3).
2. If isotretinoin has to be given, a CBC, liver function studies, and lipid profile may be indicated, along with serum or urine pregnancy tests in women.
3. Draining cysts and sinus tracts should be cultured to ensure they are not superinfected with gram-negative bacteria or coagulase-positive Staphylococcus.

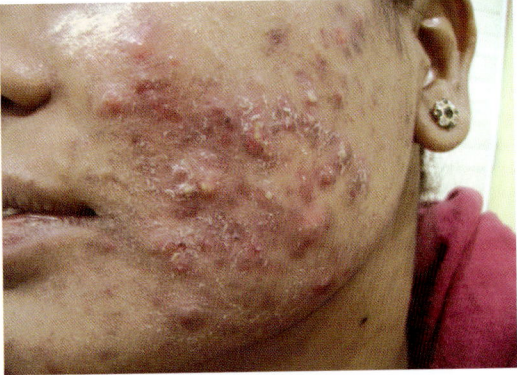

Fig. 6.3: This patient of acne conglobata was investigated and found to have a raised, free androgen index (> 6), raised prolactin, increased LH:FSH ratio

Treatment

This condition is notorious to be resistant to therapy. Thus patience and persistence, both by the physician and patient is needed to effect a complete cure.

The therapy of choice is isotretinoin 0.5–1 mg/kg for 4–6 months. Simultaneous use of systemic steroids such as prednisone 1 mg/kg/d for 2–4 weeks may also prove beneficial, particularly if systemic symptoms are evident.

Alternatives include oral tetracycline, minocycline, or doxycycline. Oral tetracycline antibiotics should not be combined with oral isotretinoin because of an increased risk of pseudotumour cerebri.

For treatment-resistant cases, dapsone 50–150 mg/d is recommended; this treatment should be carefully monitored. Treatment of acne conglobata with infliximab has been reported [Shirakawa M, 2006]. But they should be restricted for severe variants and syndromes. Because acne is part of the clinical manifestations of SAPHO, PAPA, and PASH, and because the efficacy of TNF inhibitors has been demonstrated in all 3 syndromes, it is proposed that this group of agents could be considered also in selected patients with severe primary recalcitrant acne. Off-label use of adalimumab for the treatment of AC has been reported recently [Sand FL, 2013]. Patient with facial acne conglobata have responded rapidly to treatment with etanercept [Campione E, 2006].

Reduction in weight and the stopping of smoking is important.

Procedures that may be indicated to assist with resolution of acne conglobata include aspiration of cysts/sinuses and injection of intralesional corticosteroids. Both may be performed in association with either isotretinoin or systemic antibiotic therapy, either alone or together.

Dermatological surgery with excisions of sinuses in the axillae, groin and buttocks, Z-plasty and mesh grafts or flaps are therapies restricted for the severe type of this disorder.

REFERENCES

1. Campione E, Mazzotta AM, Bianchi L, Chimenti S. Severe acne successfully treated with etanercept. Acta Derm Venereol. 2006; 86(3):256–7.

2. Chicarilli ZN.Follicular occlusion triad: Hidradenitis suppurativa, acne conglobata, and dissecting cellulitis of the scalp. Ann Plast Surg. 1987 March; 18(3):230–7.

3. Melnik B, Jansen T, Grabbe S. Abuse of anabolic-androgenic steroids and bodybuilding acne: An underestimated health problem. J Dtsch Dermatol Ges. 2007; 5(2):110–7.

4. Sand FL, Thomsen SF. Adalimumab for the treatment of refractory acne conglobata. JAMA Dermatol. 2013 Nov; 149(11):1306–7.

5. Shirakawa M, Uramoto K, Harada FA. Treatment of acne conglobata with infliximab. J Am Acad Dermatol. 2006; 55:344–6.

6. Vasanth V, Chandrashekar BS. Follicular occlusion tetrad. Indian Dermatol Online J. 2014 Oct; 5(4):491–3.

7. William J Cunliffe, Harald PM Gollnick. Acne Diagnosis and Management. Taylor and Francis. 2001.

II. ACNE EXCORIÉE

INTRODUCTION

Acne excoriée is a psychodermatological condition that refers to the behaviour of picking acne lesions [Arnold LM, 2001]. The primary pathophysiologic source is in the psyche and not in the skin. It is also known as acne excoriée des jeunes filles (excoriated acne of young girls) as it is seen more commonly in young women. It is a subset of neurotic excoriations. Acne can have a negative impact physically and psychologically, resulting in isolation and even more severe secondary impact on the psyche.

Epidemiology

Approximately 2% of the dermatology clinic patients are found to have some form of psychogenic excoriation [Bach M, 1993].

Age: The age of onset typically ranges from 15 to 45 years.

Sex: Acne excoriée is more common in females than males.

Race: Caucasian patients with acne excoriée are more common than those of African Americans or other racial groups. But no confirmatory studies of racial distribution are known.

Who Gets Acne Excoriée?

Patients with psychiatric conditions are at risk, such as:

1. *Anxiety disorders like*:
   - Generalized anxiety disorder
   - Agoraphobia
   - Panic disorder
   - Social phobia
   - Obsessive-compulsive disorder
   - Post-traumatic stress disorder [Koo J, 1995]

2. *Mood disorders*:
   - Major depression
   - Dysthymia
   - Bipolar disorders

3. *Rarely, delusional disorder* [Arnold LM, 2001].

Clinical Features

As a result of self-inflicting nature of the condition, patients tend to pick at the skin regions most easily accessible. The patients with acne excoriée can have a distribution of lesion resembling the shape of butterfly wings on the back referred to as "butterfly sign"[Koo JYM, 2003]. In this sign, there is sparing of upper, lateral sides of the back bilaterally resulting from the fact that the patient cannot reach these areas. Also, extensor aspect of the upper arm is more commonly affected than the medial aspect and more involvement of the anterior thigh than posterior thigh.

Mild acne with extensive excoriations may be present. Scar formation as a result of excoriation may be seen. Pigmentation and scars are the usual findings. Often, patients report a sense of tension immediately before picking at their skin and a sense of relief after the behavior is complete [Mancebo MC, 2011]. In some patients, no active acne lesions, only excoriations, pigmentation and scars may be seen (Fig. 6.4).

Patients can present with severe psychosocial impairment. Also, scar formation can have further negative impact, exacerbating the patients social isolation, depression and anxiety.

Diagnosis

Diagnosis is based on:
- Clinical presentation
- Detailed history
- Conducting a detailed physical examination
- Assessing patient for underlying psychiatric disorder.

Treatment

Treatment of underlying cause:
- Antidepressants with psychotherapy—it is indicated in patients with depression as the cause of acne excoriée

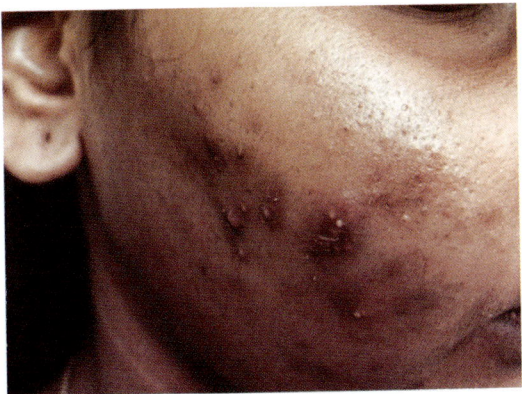

Fig. 6.4: A female patient with acne with sequelae of compulsive "picking"

- Anti-anxiolytic medication combined with psychotherapy— in patients with anxiety as the underlying cause
- Anti-OCD medication such as paroxetine and fluoxetine along with behavioural therapy—in patients with obsessive thoughts and compulsive urges to damage the skin
- selective serotonin reuptake inhibitors (SSRIs) are preferred choice for mixed depression-OCD patients, because of their dual anti-depressants and anti-OCD properties [Arnold LM, 2001].
- Behavioural therapy is more efficacious for OCD [Wilhelm S, 1999].

Treatment of hypertrophic scars and acne
- Trichloroacetic acid peels
- Skin lightening peels and also azelaic acid
- In severe cases, oral isotretinoin can be considered
- Laser treatment for scars.

REFERENCES

1. Arnold LM, Auchenbach MB, McElroy SL. Psychogenic excoriation: Clinical features, proposed diagnostic criteria, epidemiology and approaches to treatment. CNS Drugs. 2001; 15:351–9.

2. Bach M, Bach D. Psychiatric and psychometric issues in acne excoriée. Psychother Psychosom. 1993; 60:207–10.

3. Koo J. Psychodermatology: A practical manual for clinicians. Current problems in dermatology 1995; Nov/Dec: 204–32.

4. Koo JYM, Lee CS, editors. Psychocutaneous medicine. New York: Marcel Dekker; 2003.

5. Mancebo MC, Elsen JL, Sibrava NJ, Dyck IR, Rasmussen SA. Patient utilization of cognitive-behavioral therapy for OCD. Behav Ther. 2011; 42:399–412.

6. Wilhelm S, Keuthen NJ, Deckersbach T, Engelhard IM, Forker AE, Baer L, O'Sullivan RL, Jenike MA. Self-injurious skin picking: Clinical characteristics and comorbidity. J Clin Psychiatry. 1999; 60:454–9.

III. POST-ADOLESCENT FEMALE ACNE

INTRODUCTION

While acne has been traditionally considered an adolescent disorder and it was believed that most cases of acne spontaneously resolute by 25 years of age, recent trends are contrary to this view.

Indeed, the fact that the age range goes up to and occasionally beyond 45 years implies that acne is not just an adolescent problem, particularly in women, in whom the lesions are frequently perioral and occur premenstrually. In addition to the increasing incidence of post-adolescent or 'adult' acne in women, there is evidence that women are more likely than men to seek medical care for acne.

How common is it?

Cohen showed that of 51 men between the ages of 30 and 40 years, 16% of these had acne of sufficient severity to be considered clinical acne [Cibula D et al, 2000]. Cohen defined clinical acne as acne which could be seen on simple inspection without searching for it. The highest frequency of acne occurred on the chin. In the same study, an additional 121 men with clinical acne were investigated, 25% of these were over the age of 25 years and 9% were over the age of 30. As a result of these studies, the author concluded that the upper age limit of acne described by many authors was too low.

O'Loughlin attempted to classify post-adolescent acne and proposed that two subgroups existed based on examining the clinical expression of acne in 53 females, aged 24 years and over. One group suffered from continuing acne since their teenage years: This group rarely had a premenstrual flare. The second group, in contrast had no medical history or record of acne in their teenage years. Their acne appeared for the first time when they reached their 20s and in this group there were frequent occurrences of premenstrual flare-ups. After this idea was mooted there seems to be general agreement among authors, that there are individuals with continual acne from their teenage years, so called *persistent acne*, whilst for others the phenomenon is new. So-called *Late-onset* acne, which occurs after the age of 25 years.

Goulden et al. provided a detailed study of acne patients referred to an acne clinic. The mean age of patients attending the clinic was shown to have increased from 20.5 years in 1984 to 26.5 years in 1994. Further, in an investigation of 200 male and female patients over the age of 25 years, attending an acne clinic, the trunk area was most affected in males, whilst the face was the area mainly affected in women. This may explain why more females are seen in clinic for acne compared with males, despite the fact that women had a lower mean grade (0.75) for acne compared with men (1.125) on the Leeds scale. In this study, 76% of the patients seen were women. The majority of these patients had acne which had persisted from teenage years. Acne appearing for the first time after the age of 25 years (i.e. late-onset acne) was reported by 18.4% of the women and 8.3% of the men. There appeared to be no difference in the clinical presentation of persistent acne compared with late onset acne.

POSSIBLE CAUSES

There are some causes suggested, though quantification of data suggests that hormonal causes predominate.

Persistent acne could be explained as a continuation of acne occurring during teenage years and could therefore share similar pathogenic features, namely increased sebum production, ductal hypercornication, inflammation and increased bacterial activity. It is more difficult to explain *late-onset acne* which starts well after the hormonal changes accompanying puberty.

Factors put forward to explain post-adolescent acne include the use of cosmetics, stress, resistant bacteria, oral contraceptive usage, especially those with an androgenic component, and underlying hormone levels.

Androgens

Since androgens play a role in stimulating the sebaceous gland, the roles of both systemic and local tissue-derived androgens have been explored. While most women with post-adolescent acne have androgen levels in the *normal* range, several studies report lower levels of sex hormone-binding globulin (SHBG) and higher levels of free testosterone and dehydroepiandrosterone sulfate (DHEA-S) in adult female acne patients compared to controls [Aizawa H, 1993; Darley CR, 1982; Seira H, 2007; Cibula D, 2000]. However, the severity of the acne is not positively correlated with these levels. In patients with signs of hyperandrogenism, the presence of an underlying endocrine disorder such as polycystic ovarian syndrome or late-onset adrenal hyperplasia should be explored. In fact PCOS accounts for about 50% of persistent acne patients and PCOM on USG is seen in almost 80% of cases.

Our own analysis of 120 patients with persistent acne shows that, probably we are looking at the wrong markers to determine androgenicity and PCOS. Using the AMH cut off value of 3.34 ng/ ml, a definite etiology of PCOS was determined in almost 35% of cases and thus AMH should be used more often by dermatologists in diagnosing PCOS in acne patients. Also it is the peripheral androgenic conversion that is important in acne, thus 3 alpha-androstanediol glucuronide levels are more useful, than total or free testosterone.

Thus a more appropriate conclusion is that females with persistent acne are not hormonal misfits but probably have an end-organ hypersensitivity and thus blood androgen level may not be the central factor in the severity of the disease.

Adrenal Etiology

There are studies which report significantly higher levels of adrenal testosterone and DHT in adult women with acne compared with controls [Aizawa H], and congenital adrenal hyperplasia has been linked to acne. In addition, young hyperandrogenemic women with acne seem to respond abnormally to low doses of ACTH. But in our analysis of data NCCAH is not a very common cause of persistent acne.

Stress

An interesting proposition links stress to acne and is based on the premise that women with acne might have occult or hidden ovarian or adrenal dysfunction. If this is so, then these individuals could also overrespond to ACTH, triggering stress-related, adrenal androgen mediated acne [Lucky, AW]. Chronic stress activating the hypothalamic-pituitary-adrenal (HPA) axis has also been purported to exacerbate acne. Activation of HPA axis leads to both enhanced secretion of adrenal androgens and neuropeptides such as corticotrophin-releasing hormone (CRH). Recent studies demonstrate that CRH promotes lipid synthesis in the sebaceous gland and that the CRH system is abundantly expressed in acne-involved skin [Ganceviciene R, 2009].

Bacterial Resistance

Though this is a possibility, it has never been formally investigated in this population. The increase in adult acne might be related to the increasing incidence of bacteria resistant to antibiotic therapy, especially in those patients presenting persistent acne that is non-responsive to antibiotic therapy [Goulden V, 1997]. But with a rising trend of moving away from the use of antibiotics to isotretinoin, adapalene and BPO, this seems to be less likely.

In India though the situation may be different as antibiotics usage is on the rise specially the use of azithromycin, nadifloxacin and clindamycin, which can be a cause of resistance (Sardana K, 2014).

Cosmetics

Whether cosmetics are wholly or partially causative of post-adolescent acne is continually debated. In fact, at one time it was believed that cosmetic usage could be used to explain 95% of the cases of adult women presenting with a mild acneiform condition and Kligman coined the term 'acne cosmetica' to describe this persistent low-grade acne in adults.

While a variety of cosmetic ingredients are known to be comedogenic including lanolin, petrolatum, types of vegetable oils, butyl stearate, lauryl alcohol, and oleic acid, many cosmetic companies now replace these ingredients with non-comedogenic alternatives. This may be true in the West but in India, this is still not always the case. In fact a departmental analysis found that the use of various facial creams, serums and sunscreens, which are sticky and have comedogenic ingredients predispose to acne.

A study by Khanna N et al found that acne has frequently been noted in women as a direct result of facial beauty treatments. The combination of facial massage with cream, steaming and application of a face pack predisposes to acne and the the most common acne lesions were nodules, with infrequent occurrence of closed comedones.

Other Factors

Other etiological factors include genetic predisposition, smoking, and stress. The role of *heredity* in acne vulgaris is well established by several twin and cross sectional studies and the post-adolescent variant also appears to have a genetic component since 50% of patients were found to have a first-degree relative also with post-adolescent acne [Goulden V, 1997]. While the correlation between *smoking* and acne in the general population remains controversial, there appears to be a strong correlation between smoking and the comedonal post-adolescent (CPAA) variant of acne in adult females [Capitanio B, 2010]. Nicotine has been shown to have a hyperkeratizing effect by stimulating the acetylcholine receptors on epidermal keratinocytes while also being anti-inflammatory and vasoconstrictive. This correlates with the clinical picture of CPAA, a predominance of micro- and macro-comedones with a few inflammatory lesions [Misery L, 2004].

CLINICAL FEATURES

Classically post-adolescent acne has been divided into two clinical types: Persistent and late onset. Persistent acne represents a continuation of adolescent acne into adulthood. It is the more prevalent of the two types occurring in 82% of cases [Goulden et al, 1997]. Late-onset acne occurs for the first time after the age of 25 (Fig. 6.5).

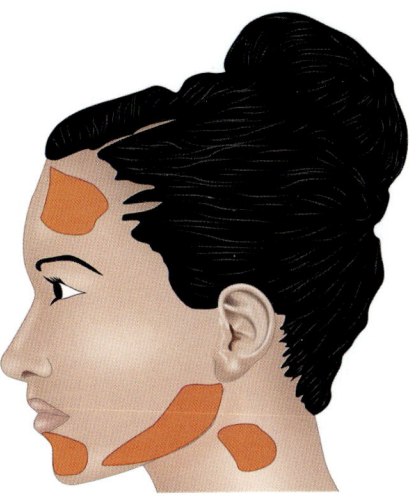

Fig. 6.5: A depiction of the sites of involvement of acne in women in persistent acne

The characteristic clinical picture for both types is mild to moderate deep-seated, tender inflammatory *papules* predominantly involving the *lower third* of the face, jaw line and neck (Fig. 6.6). The shoulders and back may also be affected. Comedonal lesions may occur on the *forehead* (Fig. 6.7) or *lateral margins* of the face but they are not prominent. Acne flares that occur premenstrually or at times of increased psychological stress are common. Several clinical variants have been described.

1. *Comedonal post-adolescent acne* (CPAA) has been documented in darker skin types (type III and IV) and is characterized by the predominance of retention lesions and micro- and macrocomedones,

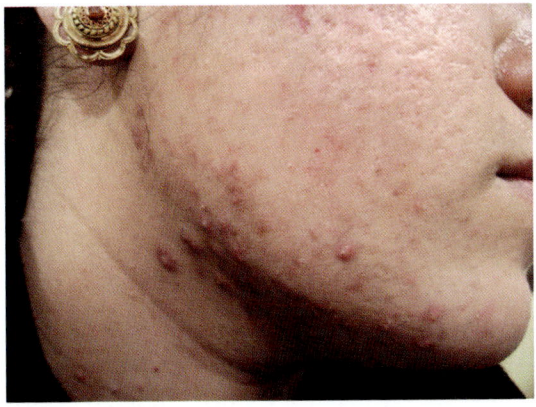

Fig. 6.6: A female patient with PCOS with acne along the jaw line

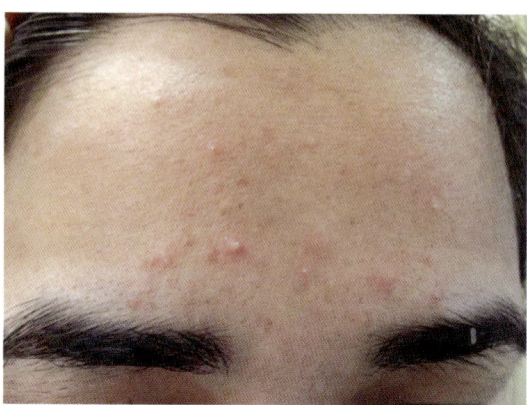

Fig. 6.7: An uncommon presentation with forehead involvement of acne in post-adolscent female

with fewer than 5% inflammatory lesions. The comedones are homogenously distributed over the entire face [Capitanio B, 2010]. While acne scarring is usually attributed to inflammatory lesions, ice pick scars occur in CPAA patients, and in severe cases numerous ice pick scars can coalesce into craters.

2. *Chin acne* is a clinical variant in mature females, which is characterized by premenstrual flares of inflammatory papules on the chin and perioral region (Fig. 6.8).

3. *Sporadic acne:* This consists of unpredictable sudden outbreaks of inflammatory papules and pustules in usually one but sometimes several locations in middle-aged and older adults. These outbreaks usually coincide with a systemic illness or surgical operation, although inciting events are not always found [Marks R, 2004].

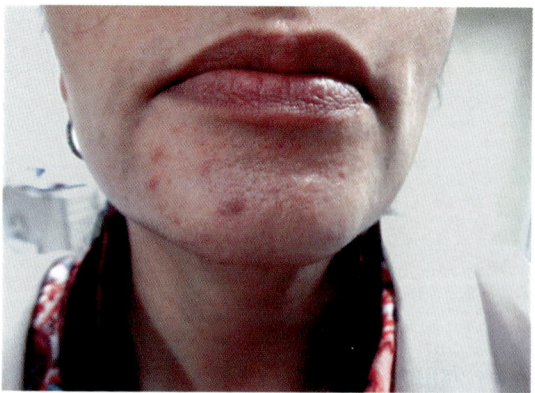

Fig. 6.8: This patient had involvement of the chin. She had no biochemical problem but responded to spironolactone 100 mg

INVESTIGATIONS

Though routine investigation are not advisable there are two situations where this is useful. First is the patient who failed therapy, specially isotretinoin. Second are patients with features of hyperandrogenism, including irregular menses, hirsutism, alopecia, infertility, deepening of voice, increased libido, acanthosis nigricans, and truncal obesity. Features of hyperandrogenism are not uncommon in adult female acne patients, occurring in 37 % [Goulden et al, 1997] of patients, and should be sought out by a focused medical history and physical examination (Fig. 6.9)

Polycystic ovarian syndrome (PCOS) is the most common cause of hyperandrogenism in women and is important to be identified since it may impart an increased risk for type 2 diabetes mellitus and cardiovascular disease (Fig. 6.10).

The screening laboratory tests for an underlying endocrine disorder consist of serum DHEA-S, total testosterone, free testosterone, and luteinizing hormone/follicle-stimulating hormone (LH/FSH) ratio and are detailed in the chapter on investigations. Since the hormone surge that occurs with ovulation can cause an inaccurate assessment, these tests should be drawn either just before or during the menstrual period (day 3). Oral contraceptives may mask underlying hyperandrogenism, therefore the oral contraceptives should be discontinued 4–6 weeks prior to laboratory assessment.

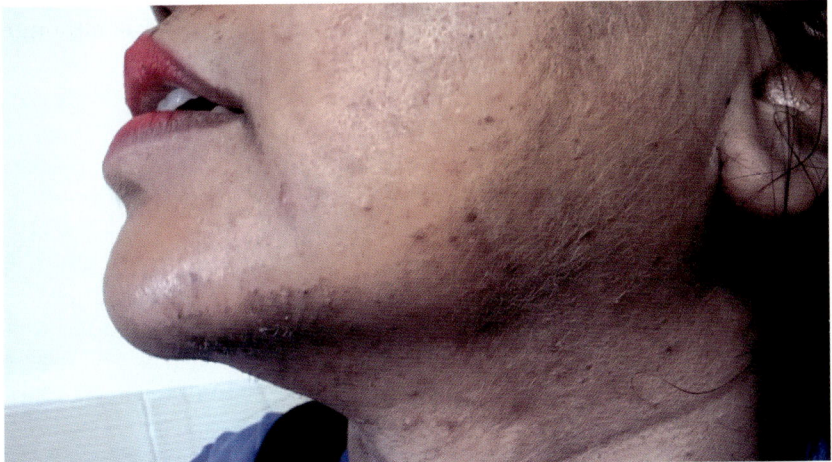

Fig. 6.9: This patient has hirsutism with "jaw line" acne. The patient had a deranged androgen index (12.3) and was put on OCP plus spironolactone and low dose isotretinoin

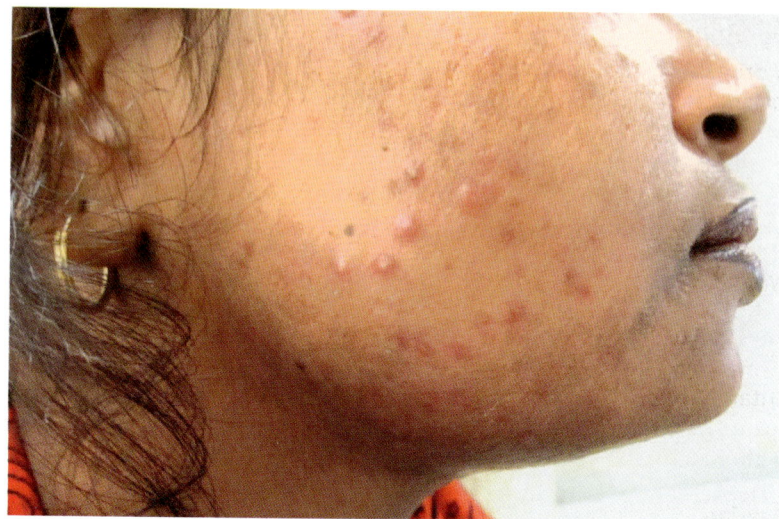

Fig. 6.10: A case of acne with hirsutism, the patient also was a diagnosed case of PCOS

TREATMENT

The general principles of treating female post-adolescent acne are not significantly different from treating other acne populations, as in most cases the cause is the same.

Older skin tends to be more sensitive to the potential irritant effects of topical retinoids but more resistant to the irritant effects of benzoyl peroxide [Marks R, 2004], which is good as BPO has a high efficacy rate and is also helpful in preventing resistance.

Acne is a chronic condition for many of these patients with 81% of women reporting failures with systemic antibiotics and 15–30% having had recurrence after isotretinoin treatment [Ebede TL, 2009]. Hormonal therapies can be a useful therapeutic approach and can be effective even in patients with normal serum androgen levels [Thiboutot D, 2004]. This is detailed in a previous chapter and a summary is given Table 6.1.

My approach is to combine a OCP (drosperinone combination) or spironolactone with existing acne therapy. It must be understood that hormonal therapy is not useful as a monotherapy. If it is given as a monotherapy an average of 3–6 months of therapy is required before an appreciable result is achieved.

Table 6.1 *Summary of antiandrogens used in hormonal acne*

Androgen receptor blockers

Spironolactone	50–200 mg daily	Menstrual irregularities, breast tenderness, hyperkalemia, birth defects, hypotension, headache, dizziness, downiness, confusion, nausea, vomiting, anorexia, diarrhoea
Cyproterone acetate	50–100 mg daily or 2 mg with 35 µg of ethinyl estradiol	Breast tenderness, headache, nausea, breakthrough bleeding, fatal hepatotoxicity, birth defects
Flutamide	62.5–500 mg daily	Breast-tenderness, gastrointestinal upset, hot flushes, decreased libido, fatal hepatitis, birth defects

Ovarian androgen production blocker

Oral contraceptives	**EE(µg)/progesterone (mg)**
	30/Drospirenone 3 (DRONIS 30*)
	20/Drospirenone 3 (DRONIS 20)
	20/Desogestrel 0.15 mg (FEMILON)
	35/Cyproterone 2 (Diane-35)

Adrenal androgen production blocker

Glucocorticoids	2.5–5 mg daily (HS)

*FDA approved in acne

REFERENCES

1. Aizawa H, Niimura M. Adrenal androgen abnormalities in women with late onset and persistent acne. Arch Dermatol Res. 1993; 284:451–5.
2. Capitanio B, Sinagra JL, Bordignon V, Cordiali Fei P, Picardo M, Zouboulis CC. Underestimated clinical features of post-adolescent acne. J Am Acad Dermatol. 2010; 63:782–8.
3. Cibula D, Hill M, Vohradnikova O, Kuzel D, Fanta M, Zivny J. The role of androgens in determining acne severity in adult women. Br J Dermatol. 2000; 143:399–404.
4. Cohen, E.L. Incidence of clinical acne in man. Lancet 1, 168 (1942).
5. Darley CR, Kirby JD, Besser GM et al. Circulating testosterone, sex hormone binding globulin and prolactin in women with late onset or persistent acne vulgaris . Br J Dermatol. 1982 May; 106(5):517–22.
6. Ebede TL, Arch EL, Berson D. Hormonal treatment of acne in women. J Clin Aesthetic Dermatol. 2009; 2:16–22.
7. Goulden V, Clark SM, Cunliffe WJ. Post-adolescent acne: A review of clinical features. Br J Dermatol. 1997; 136:66–70.

8. Ganceviciene R, Graziene V, Fimmel S, Zouboulis CC. Involvement of the corticotropin-releasing hormone system in the pathogenesis of acne vulgaris. Br J Dermatol. 2009; 160:345–52.

9. Khanna, N. and Gupta, S.D. Acneiform eruptions after facial beauty treatment. Int. J. Dermatol. 38, 196–199 (1999).

10. Kligman, A.M. and Mills, O.H. Acne cosmetica. Arch. Dermatol. 111, 65–68 (1975).

11. Lucky, A.W., Rosenfield, R.L., McGuire, J. et al. Adrenal androgen hyperresponsiveness to adrenocorticotropin women with acne and/or hirsutism: Adrenal enzyme defects and exaggerated adrenarche. J. Clin. Endocrinol. Metab. 62, 840–848 (1986).

12. Marks R. Acne and its management beyond the age of 35 years. Am J Clin Dermatol. 2004; 5:459–62.

13. Misery L. Nicotine effects on the skin: Are they positive or negative? Exp Dermatol. 2004; 13:665–70.

14. O'Loughlin, M. Acne in the adult female. Aust. J. Dermatol. 7, 218–222 (1964).

15. Sardana K, Garg VK. Antibiotic resistance in acne: is it time to look beyond antibiotics and *Propionobacterium acnes*? Int J Dermatol. 2014 Jul; 53(7):917–9.

16. Seirafi H, Farnaghi F, Vasheghani-Farahani A, et al. Assessment of androgens in women with adult-onset acne. Int J Dermatol. 2007; 46:1188–91.

17. Thiboutot D. Acne: Hormonal concepts and therapy. Clin Dermatol. 2004; 22:419–28.

IV. POST-INFLAMMATORY PIGMENT ALTERATION

INTRODUCTION

Acne vulgaris (AV) in skin of colour is similar to acne anywhere else in the world except the almost invariable degree of post-inflammatory hyperpigmentation (PIH) (Fig. 6.11). PIH is often of equal or greater concern to patients with skin of colour as the acne itself. Patients frequently refer to the lesions of PIH as scars, and the cosmetic disfigurement caused by PIH adds to the psychological distress associated with acne.

While pigmentary alterations can occur without manipulation of acne lesions, they tend to be more severe and of longer duration in excoriated lesions (e.g. in patients with acne excoriée). Excoriated lesions typically appear as hypopigmented macules with hyperpigmented borders.

However, it is important to keep in mind that in addition to acne itself, various acne treatments can cause hyper- or hypopigmentation as a result of irritation.

Why does PIH Happen?

A key characteristic in skin of colour is the tendency for melanocytes to exhibit labile responses to inflammation and injury [Ruiz-Maldonado R, 1997; Grimes PE, 2009], which contributes to the high prevalence of post-inflammatory hyperpigmentation in darker skin types. Inflammatory mediators, including prostaglandins and leukotrienes, can stimulate increased melanin synthesis, which can lead to increased pigment in the epidermis alone or also in the dermis [Grimes PE, 1999]. When there is dermal involvement, there is disruption of the basal layer that leads to macrophages engulfing the

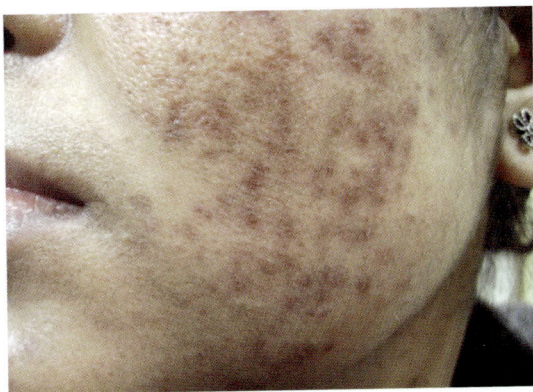

Fig. 6.11: A female patient with persistent pigmentation following healing of acne lesions

melanin and the formation of melanophages. A study by Halder *et al.* examined biopsies in thirty black patients with acne vulgaris and found the presence of inflammation histologically even in clinically non-inflammatory lesions such as comedones. In addition, papules and pustules displayed considerable inflammation histologically that extended significantly beyond the margins of each lesion. While subclinical inflammation is likely a feature of acne vulgaris in all skin types, it may contribute to the tendency toward dyschromias in acne patients with skin of colour.

Clinical Presentation

Post-inflammatory hyperpigmentation (PIH) from acneiform lesions appears as macules or patches of darker skin colour in contrast to the patient's natural skin colour (Fig. 6.12). With dermal deposition of melanin, the duration of the hyperpigmentation is prolonged and can last several months to years. Hypopigmentation can also be seen in acne patients as a sequela of irritant dermatitis from topical acne therapies. It can also be seen with the use of skin lightening agents to lighten PIH, typically presenting with perilesional halos of hypopigmentation.

In India, combination of BPO >5% and sulphur and use of steroids can add to the issue of PIH and hypopigmentation.

Treatment

Some general principles are given below, though some of them like sunscreens use may be a double-edged sword as using the wrong base can actually cause acne!

1. Sun Protection

One of the hallmarks of post-inflammatory hyperpigmentation management is sun protection with broad-spectrum sunscreens

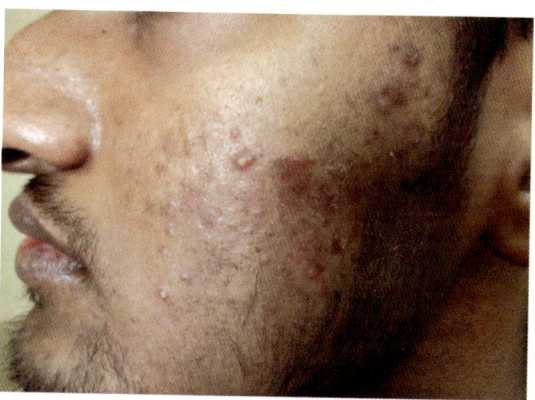

Fig. 6.12: A male case with acne healing with pigmentation

including physical blockers to prevent both ultraviolet and visible light induced melanogenesis as well as wearing wide-brimmed hats and adhering to overall sun avoidance. This is important in our skin type my preference is for mat-based or silicone-based sunscreens. Lotions and hydrogels can be sticky and predispose to acne. Another option is to use a concealer or a light foundation as they itself act as a sunscreen. Ironically in India, those who can afford sunscreens are in office jobs and those who cannot are in the sun, thus a simple advise is to avoid direct sun exposure between 11 am and 3 pm!

2. Topical Agents

A. Hydroquinone

The efficacy of hydroquinone (HQ), a first-line therapy for hyperpigmentation for close to 50 years, is a useful tool in acne, though excessive use can lead to a risk of a "halo" of hypopigmentation on perilesional skin. Also irritant contact dermatitis (which must be monitored closely as this can potentiate post-inflammatory pigment alteration), and rarely exogenous ochronosis can be seen.

B. Retinoids

Proposed mechanisms of topical retinoids for the improvement of hyperpigmentation include inhibition of tyrosinase induction in melanocytes, enhancement of desquamation that speed up sloughing of melanin in keratinocytes, inhibition of melanosome transfer from melanocytes to keratinocytes, allowing greater penetration of other active ingredients, and redistribution or dispersion of epidermal melanin [Ortonne JP, 2006]. Clinicians must also be aware of the potential of topical retinoids to induce irritation that could also potentially potentiate post-inflammatory pigment alteration. Thus gentler agents like adapalene and tretinoin microspheres should be used than tazarotene and non-micronized tretinoin.

C. Combination creams

Studies of dual or triple agent combination therapies that may include a topical retinoid, hydroquinone, and a topical corticosteroid in comparison to single agents have shown to be more effective with a more rapid response in pigment disorders.

In a multicentred, investigator blinded, randomized study of 792 patients with post-inflammatory hyperpigmentation secondary to acne vulgaris that compared triple combination cream (fluocinolone acetonide 0.01%, hydroquinone 4%, and tretinoin 0.05%) to each of its dyads, results indicated more patients treated with triple therapy for 8 weeks achieved clear or almost clear status than any of the dyad comparators [Baumann L, 2007]. In India though the real worry is of misuse of such creams, which can over a longer period of time can actually cause acne.

Other therapeutic considerations for dyschromia include products containing azelaic acid, kojic acid and glycolic acid.

Cosmeceuticals have become increasingly popular for consumers interested in hyperpigmentation remedies. Certain ingredients in these products are popular including soy, liquiritin (licorice extract), N-acetylglucosamine, niacinamide, mequinol (4-hydroxyanisole), vitamin C (ascorbic acid), oligopeptide, rucinol, tranexamic acid, and N-undecyl-10-enoyl-1-phenylalanine [Sardana K, 2015]. Products that include soy or nicotinamide prevent melanosome transfer [Sardana K], while hydroquinone, arbutin, licorice, azelaic acid, and kojic acid inhibit tyrosinase [Sardana K, 2015]. Newer combination formulations such as emblica, kojic acid, and glycolic acid (skinceuticals); lipo-hydroxy acid, glycolic acid, and kojic acid (La Roche-Posay); and kojic acid, licorice extract, and vitamin C (neostrata) may also be useful adjuncts to the treatment of PIH. Potential emerging products for pigment disorders include grape seed extract, ellagic acid, linoleic acid, aleosin, green tea extracts, and lignin peroxidase [Sardana K, 2015]. As a thumb rule they are inferior in action to HQ and thus are a gentle method to remove PIH.

D. Azelaic acid

Azelaic acid 20% cream has also been found to successfully treat acne. It has been reported to be as effective as tretinoin 0.05% cream, BPO 5% gel, erythromycin 2% ointment, and clindamycin 1% gel [Gollnick HP, 2004; Webster G, 2000] . It is not only an anti-inflammatory agent but also reduces *P. acnes* proliferation and normalizes keratinization. Like BPO, *P. acnes* resistance to azelaic acid has not been reported [Webster G, 2000]. Azelaic acid is well tolerated and relatively mild, so it is a suitable option for individuals with sensitive skin [Callender VD, 2004]. It appears to have an inhibitory effect on melanocyte proliferation and melanogenesis, so it can potentially reduce hyperpigmentation [Sardana K, 2015].

It is an especially useful treatment option for skin of colour patients with PIH who cannot tolerate retinoids. Azelaic acid can be combined with other acne therapies to improve efficacy.

The issue is of the base, thus the cream base can be used for dry skin and the gel base for oily skin. The lotion form is better and I feel that azelaic acid is the perfect agent to tackle acne and PIH, though it may not be effective as BPO, in terms of the onset of action.

E. Cosmetic procedures

While topical therapies are usually the initial approach to the treatment of post-inflammatory hyperpigmentation, physical therapies, such as chemical peels and microdermabrasion, may also be used as adjuncts to improve treatment outcomes.

Superficial chemical peels such as salicylic acid (20–30%), glycolic acid (20–70%), trichloroacetic acid [TCA] (10–25%), and Jessner's solution as an adjunctive approach with topical agents may help improve hyperpigmentation by removing excess epidermal melanin and enhancing penetration of topical bleaching agents [Briganti S, 2003].

Various studies have reported that the addition of serial glycolic acid chemical peels to a topical regimen is beneficial for the treatment of hyperpigmentation from melasma with a trend toward more rapid and greater improvement [Javaheri SM, 2001; Sarkar R, 2002], and this approach can similarly be applied to post-inflammatory hyper-pigmentation. Burns *et al.* specifically studied this hyperpigmentation in 19 patients with darker skin and found a trend toward more rapid and greater improvement when six serial glycolic acid peels were added to a topical regimen of 2% hydroquinone/10% glycolic acid gel twice daily as well as tretinoin 0.05% cream at bedtime in comparison to those who only maintained the topical regimen without receiving the chemical peels.

In regard to serial salicylic acid peels, a study of 35 Korean patients receiving 30% salicylic acid peels biweekly for 12 weeks found this to be a safe and effective therapy for acne in Asian patients [Lee HS, 2003]. There are multiple studies on salicylic acid peels in the treatment of post-inflammatory hyperpigmentation [Grimes PE, 1999, Ahn HH, 2006; Joshi SS, 2009], but sadly in India there are no well conducted studies on this peel in acne patients. It is my opinion that being a non-inflammatory peel and ideal for lipid rich skin with an excellent comedolytic potential and penetration into the sebum rich follicle salicylic acid is the ideal peel for acne patients. With glycolic acid, the titration has to be perfect and it is an inflammatory peel and can induce PIH in cases if not done properly.

F. Lasers

While there is an increasing amount of literature on chemical peels for dyschromias, there is limited literature on photodynamic and other light-/laser-based therapies in the management of post-inflammatory hyperpigmentation.

Lasers are *unpredictable* in the treatment of hyperpigmentation and therefore are usually reserved for failures of combination topical

Table 6.2 *Treatment pearls for acne in SOC* (Sejal K Shah)*

Reduce inflammation
- Initiate effective and appropriately aggressive treatment early in disease course
- Include topical BPO (micronized) and topical retinoid (micronized) in treatment regimen
- Low threshold to initiate oral antibiotics when indicated
- Topical BPO/clindamycin or azelaic acid is a good way of tackling both acne and PIH
- Low dose isotretinoin is another good option

Minimize irritation
- Avoid sulphur, gylcolic acid
- Appropriate selection of vehicle, concentration, and dosing. Alcohol based agents should be avoided

Eliminate exacerbating factors
- Use silicone-based hair products and noncomedogenic cosmetics (e.g. mineral make ups) and moisturizers

Avoid steroid use on the face

Educate patient about PIH
- Difference between active acne lesions and PIH
- Establish realistic expectation regarding treatment outcome (e.g. length of treatment, potential need for adjunctive treatments for PIH)
- Importance of sun protection (sunscreens with the wrong base can actually cause acne)

*SOC: Skin of colour

therapy and chemical peels. If considered, skin type should always be taken into account given the high risk of post-inflammatory hyper-pigmentation (Table 6.2).

While fractional nonablative lasers may be useful for hyper-pigmentation, optimal treatment parameters for dyschromias in skin of colour have not been well established and treatment outcomes are unpredictable; however, lower treatment levels and prophylactic use of hydroquinone both before and after laser treatment are recommended to minimize post-treatment hyperpigmentation.

SUMMARY

PIH is a major issue in Indian patients. Even amongst experts there is a variation in diagnosis of PIH, specially when active acne was present. Thus PIH is a issue which should be tackled at the very outset.

I believe that three agents are excellent for PIH, one is low dose isotretinoin, that prevents acne and peels of the skin, salicylic acid gel 2% and time! I do not believe that HQ can do anything marked specially after the PIH has occurred. Most importantly I follow the *NO STEROID ON THE FACE POLICY*. It does more harm than good as it delays the healing and can itself cause atrophy. A list of common sense options are given below for a quick reference, but as a thumb rule the less you irritate the skin, lesser the PIH.

REFERENCES

1. Ahn HH, Kim IH. Whitening effect of salicylic acid peels in Asian patients. Dermatol Surg. 2006;32(3):372–5. PubMed PMID: 16640681. discussion 5. Epub 2006/04/28. eng.

2. Baumann L, Grimes P, Pandya AG, et al. Triple combination cream is an effective treatment for post-inflammatory hyperpigmentation. Presented at the 65th Annual American Academy of Dermatology Conference, Washington, DC, 3–5 Feb 2007.

3. Briganti S, Camera E, Picardo M. Chemical and instrumental approaches to treat hyperpigmentation. Pigment Cell Res. 2003; 16(2):101–10.

4. Burns RL, Prevost-Blank PL, Lawry MA, Lawry TB, Faria DT, Fivenson DP. Glycolic acid peels for postinflammatory hyperpigmentation in black patients. A comparative study. Dermatol Surg. 1997; 23(3):171–4.

5. Callender VD. Acne in ethnic skin: Special considerations for therapy. Dermatol Ther. 2004; 17(2):184–95.

6. Gollnick HP, Graupe K, Zaumseil RP. Azelaic acid 15% gel in the treatment of acne vulgaris. Combined results of two double-blind clinical comparative studies. J Dtsch Dermatol Ges. 2004; 2(10):841–7.

7. Grimes PE. Management of hyperpigmentation in darker racial ethnic groups. Semin Cutan Med Surg. 2009 Jun;28(2):77–85.

8. Grimes PE. The safety and efficacy of salicylic acid chemical peels in darker racial-ethnic groups. Dermatol Surg. 1999; 25(1):18–22.

9. Halder R, Holmes Y, Bridgeman-Shah S, Kligman A. A clinical pathological study of acne vulgaris in black females. J Invest Dermatol. 1996; 106(4):888. 2009; 28(2):77–85.

10. Javaheri SM, Handa S, Kaur I, Kumar B. Safety and efficacy of glycolic acid facial peel in Indian women with melasma. Int J Dermatol. 2001; 40(5):354–7.

11. Joshi SS, Boone SL, Alam M, Yoo S, White L, Rademaker A, et al. Effectiveness, safety, and effect on quality of life of topical salicylic acid peels for treatment of post-inflammatory hyperpigmentation in dark skin. Dermatol Surg. 2009; 35(4):638–44.

12. Lee HS, Kim IH. Salicylic acid peels for the treatment of acne vulgaris in Asian patients. Dermatol Surg. 2003; 29(12):1196–9.

13. Ortonne JP. Retinoid therapy of pigmentary disorders. Dermatol Ther. 2006; 19(5):280–8.

14. Ruiz-Maldonado R, Orozco-Covarrubias ML. Post-inflammatory hypopigmentation and hyperpigmentation. Semin Cutan Med Surg. 1997; 16(1):36–43.

15. Sardana K, Ghunawat S. Rationale of using hypopigmenting drugs and their clinical application in melasma. Expert Rev Clin Pharmacol. 2015 Jan; 8(1):123–34.

16. Sarkar R, Kaur C, Bhalla M, Kanwar AJ. The combination of glycolic acid peels with a topical regimen in the treatment of melasma in dark-skinned patients: A comparative study. Dermatol Surg. 2002; 28(9): 828–32.

17. Sejal K. Shah and Andrew F. Alexis. Acne and Rosacea in Skin of Color. Skin of Color: A Practical Guide to Dermatologic Diagnosis and Treatment, DOI 10.1007/978-0-387-84929-4_2, ©Springer Science+Business Media New York 2013.

18. Webster G. Combination azelaic acid therapy for acne vulgaris. J Am Acad Dermatol. 2000; 43(2 Pt 3):S47–50.

V. HORMONAL ACNE

INTRODUCTION

Acne vulgaris is the most common skin condition treated by physicians worldwide. Hormonal acne is a term loosely used to refer to those acne where various hormones act as a major influence in their pathogenesis, making them *persistent* and *therapy* resistant. Hormonal acne may or may not have obvious cutaneous signs or biochemical evidence of hyperandrogenism [Cunliffe *et al*, 2009]. For such endocrinal pathogenic acne, hormonal therapy is the logical therapeutic solution. But hormonal therapy is not strictly indicated for only those acne patients who have cutaneous or biochemical evidence of hyper-androgenism, rather it can be used even *without* any evidence of hyperandrogenism, for therapy resistant acne [Bhambri *et al*, 2009]. They can be prescribed as monotherapy but when used in combination with other conventional therapy, they may prove to be more beneficial [Simpson *et al*, 2004]. Hormonal evaluation is a prerequisite for hormonal therapy, to identify the cause behind hyperandrogenism, which may be ovarian or adrenal.

Clinical Features

For acne vulgaris, the peak incidence is seen between 14 and 17 years in girls and 16 and 19 years in boys. The condition principally affects the face, chest and back, which have a high density of sebaceous gland.

Hormonal acne will also present in similar manner without much variation in clinical presentation (Fig. 6.13). Clinically, patients with hormone related acne can be recognized by the concentration of lesions along the *jaw line and chin* (Fig. 6.14) [Harper JC, 2006].

A suspicion for hormonal background for acne and need for a hormonal analysis should be reserved for therapy resistant, relapsing, [George R, 2008] or late onset (after 35 years of age) [Harper JC, 2006], prepubertal, stress or prementruation exaggerbated acne [Goulden *et al*, 1997], if associated signs of hyperandrogenism like hirsutism androgenetic alopecia, seborrhoea are

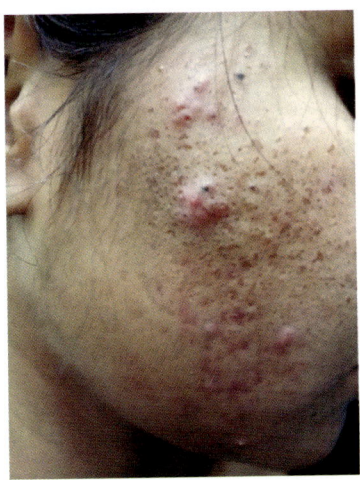

Fig. 6.13: Clinical presentation of acne in a 36 years old lady with hyperandrogenemia

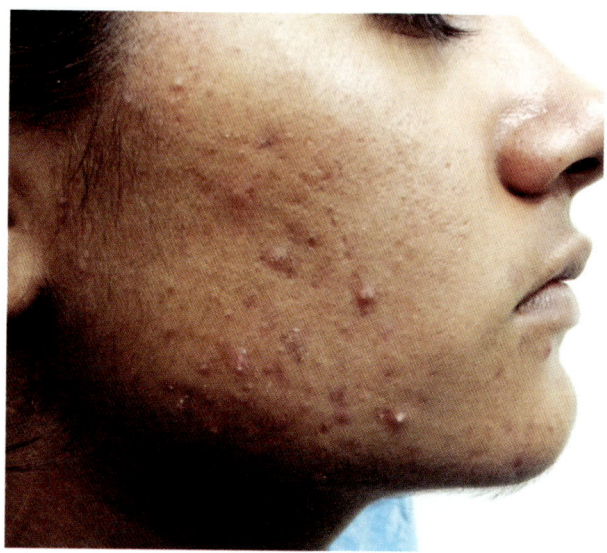

Fig. 6.14: Distribution of acne lesions along the jaw line in a 40-year-old lady

present[7] [George R, 2008], in patients of PCOD (polycystic ovarian disease) [Gollnick *et al*, 2003], SAHA syndrome (seborrhoea, acne, hirsutism and androgenetic alopecia) [Gollnick *et al*, 2003], HAIR-AN syndrome (hyperandrogenism, insulin resistance and acanthosis nigricans) [Gollnick *et al*, 2003], and in patients with associated signs of virilizations like male body contour, deep voice, cliteromegaly and hirsutism, etc. [Jacqueline M, 2010]

Endocrinal Causes

Various hormones that can influence acnegenesis are:

a. *Androgens:* Increased sebum production due to androgens activity at the sebaceous follicle is a prerequisite for acne in all patients. High level of androgens, or hypersensitivity of the sebaceous glands to a normal level of androgens, causes an increase in sebum production [Jacqueline M, 2010; Pochi, 1982; Pochi PE, 1990]. In addition, androgens may also enhance follicular hyperkeratosis independent of their effect on the sebaceous glands. Zona reticularis in adrenal cortex and theca lutein cells in mature follicle in ovaries are the predominant sites where androgen production takes place. Androgenic hormones include strong androgen, which is testosterone, and weaker androgens like androstenedione and dehydroepiandrostenedione (DHEA). Weak androgens like androstenedione and DHEA get converted to testosterone in peripheral tissues like adipose tissue, muscle and skin. Finally, testosterone gets coverted to dihydrotestosterone by 5α-reductase before it binds androgen receptors in target tissues [Pochi PE, 1990].

b. *Progesterone:* Progesterone is a competitive inhibitor of 5α reductase and might be expected to reduce gland activity. The fluctuation of sebum production in women during menstrual cycle and premenstrual flare has partly been blamed on progesterone [Klingman *et al*, 1958].

c. *Estrogen:* Estrogen, in high doses, decreases the size of sebaceous gland and reduce sebum production by reducing endogenous androgen production via a negative feedback effect on the pituitary gonadal axis [Pochi *et al*, 1995].

d. *Insulin:* High level of insulin and IGF-1 increases production of sebum. They promote androgen synthesis in ovaries by helping theca cells to escape desensitization to high level of LH. IGFs, IGF-binding protein 3 have been implicated in acnegenesis [Ehrmann *et al*, 1995]

e. *Adrenocortical hormones:* Glucocorticoids stimulate sebocytes proliferation. Hydrocortisone given to prepubertal boys cause enlargement of sebaceous glands [Chen *et al*, 2002].

Apart from these above mentioned hormones a few pituitary hormones like adrenocorticotropic hormone (ACTH), growth hormones (GH), luteinizing hormone (LH) and prolactin can also have some influencing affect on acne pathogenesis [Schmidt *et al*, 1991; Beylot *et al*, 1998].

Investigation

For patients with cutaneous hyperandrogenism, hormonal evaluation is a prerequisite for hormonal therapy. The patient should be off any oral contraceptives or any other hormonal therapy for at least one month before testing and the tests should be performed at the onset of menses (luteal phase) [Jacqueline M, 2010] and the hormones that need to be investigated for are:

a. *Testosterone (free and total):* If there is only a modest elevation of total testosterone but it remains <200 ng/dl, probably, it is probably due to a benign pathology such as PCOS or adrenal hyperplasia. But beyond this level, one should suspect androgen secreting neoplasia of either ovaries or adrenals [Lin-Su, 2008]. Notably in females with persistent acne high normal levels are often seen.

b. *Androstenedione:* Androstenedione secretion follows a circadian rhythm and has its peak in the morning, hence, early morning sample between 0700 and 0900 hours should be measured. Androstenedione is normally secreted equally from both ovaries and adrenals [Bhambri *et al*, 2009]. In acne patients there is no significant difference in androstenedione levels between patients and controls

c. *Dehydroepiandrosterone (DHEA):* 90% of DHEA and 98% of dehydroepiandrosterone sulfate (DHEAS) are secreted from zona reticularis of adrenal cortex. Hence elevated level of DHEA and its sulfate points towards an adrenal source. Modest elevation of DHEAS (4000–8000 ng/dL) may indicate benign adrenal hyperplasia, while higher levels should prompt evaluation for an adrenal tumour [Lin-Su *et al,* 2008; Eric *et al,* 2001].

d. *SHBG:* If SHBG level in blood decreases, then free testosterone level in blood goes up resulting in a state of relative hyperandrogenism [Eric *et al,* 2001]. Abnormalities of serum androgens and sex hormone binding globulin (SHBG) alone or in combination can be seen leading to a elevation in the Free Androgen Index. A study (Darley CR) found that abnormalities of serum androgens and sex hormone binding globulin (SHBG) alone or in combination were present in 52% of the patients. Elevated serum testosterone and low SHBG were the commonest abnormalities found (46%). *17-OH-Progesterone:* Thuis is elevated(>200 ng/dl) in CAH or NCAH, because when there is deficiency or absence of 21α *hydroxylase,* the pathways dedicated for aldosterone and cortisol synthesis get blocked and androgen secretion pathway gets accelerated [Lin-Su *et al,* 2008]. But any diagnosis of NCCAH should be confirmed by using the ACTH stimulation test

e. *LH : FSH:* A ratio of >3 is seen in PCOS patients [Chang *et al,* 1999].

f. *Prolactin:* Prolactin would be raised due to hyperprolactinemia (in hypothalamic disease or a pituitary tumour). [Schmidt, 1991. But in acne in most cases this is usually normal.

g. *Serum cortisol:* In adrenal neoplasia, all layers of adrenal cortex may be hyperactive resulting in a cushingoid status.

h. *Fasting and postprandial insulin:* In presence of cutaneous markers for hyperinsulinemia, serum level of insulin should be measured to rule out hyperinsulinemia which is an important association of PCOS and independently also can play a hormonal role in acne genesis [Ehrmann *et al,* 1995].

To confirm the source of excess androgen, one should either do an ACTH stimulation test or a dexamethasone suppression test. Ovarian source of excess androgen will fail to respond to this test whereas the adrenal androgen level would increase following ACTH stimulation and decrease following dexamethasone suppression test [Thiboutot D, 2001]. Imaging studies like ultrasound ovaries (preferably performed in luteal phase) and adrenals are recommended to look for any mass or cyst and CT/MRI for further delineation of the mass, if there is any.

It must be pointed that except in cases of an overt underlying disorder like PCOS, there is little correlation of the androgen levels and the severity, distribution or pattern of acne or the presence of hirsuties or irregular periods. But even in the patients with no lab abnormalities there is a possibility of end organ sensitivity, thus antiandrogens are of potential use.

Treatment

Most of the hormonal therapies are mainly directed at suppressing ovarian or adrenal sources of androgens or blocking activation and action of androgens in sebaceous gland and probably follicular keratinocytes as well. This can be accomplished by using the following:

1. *Suppressors of Ovarian Androgen Secretion*

a. *Oral contraceptives (OCs):* Estrogen, i.e. ethinyl estradiol (EE) suppresses the ovarian production of androgens by suppressing gonadotropin release from hypothalamus via a negative feedback effect. They also stimulate hepatic synthesis of SHBG, and inhibit 5α *reductase* activity [Arowojolu *et al*, 2009]. Low dose estrogen (EE 0.020–0.050 µg) is usually combined with various progestins (Levonorgesterol, Desogestrel, Norgestimate and Gestodene), to avoid the risk of endometrial cancer associated with unopposed estrogens [Lucky, 1997; Rothman, 1993]. It is administered from day-1 of menstrual cycle and given in 21 days on 7 days off regimen, after obtaining a negative pregnancy report. Common side-effects, which usually subside after 2 to 3 months, are breakthrough bleeding, nausea, breast tenderness and weight gain. Less common side effects include decreased libido, melasma, mood changes. More serious side effects like stroke and heart attacks are minimal with the newer OCs. Contraindications to OCs use are pregnancy, lactation, poorly controlled hypertention, angina, complicated valvular disease, coagulation disorders, personal or family history of thrombotic disorders, severe obesity, undiagnosed uterine bleeding or estrogen dependent neoplasm, neurological symptoms, hepatic dysfunction, etc [Lucky *et al*, 1997; Harper JC, 2009].

Dermatologists can initiate an OC prescription with an advice to follow up with a gynaecologist because a physical examination, including a pelvic examination might be appropriate. Apart from the decreased androgen level, other additional benefits of OCs in acne patients are contraception, which is advised along with isotretinoin therapy and menstrual irregularities too respond positively with OCs [Harper JC 2009]. In a recent publication, it was stated that concomitant use of antibiotics such as tetracycline, doxycycline, with OCs do not interfere with contraceptive steroid levels [Murphy *et al*, 1991]. Example of a few such OCs available in Indian market are *Crisanta* (EE 0.03 mg + Drospirenone 3 mg), *Femilon* (EE 0.02 mg + Desogestrel 0.15 mg), *Yasmin* (EE 0.03 mg + 3 mg Drospirenone). Although effects of OCs as monotherapy have been well established, they should always be used in combination with other topical and oral therapies for acne for better result [Haroun M, 2004].

b. *Cyproterone acetate (CPA)*: Cyproterone acetate is a progestational anti-androgen that also blocks androgen receptors. Overall improvement of 75–90% has been reported in patients treated with CPA 50 to 100 mg daily (with or without EE) [Vas Wayjen, 1995; Gollnick, 1999]. In India, CPA is available in combination with EE (e.g. Diane 35). Side effects include menstrual abnormalities, breast tenderness and enlargement, nausea/ vomiting, fluid retention, leg edema, headache, liver dysfunction and rarely blood clotting disorders [Hammerstein *et al*, 1975].

c. *Gonadotropin releasing hormone (GnRH) analogues*: GnRH analogues inhibit ovarian androgen production by blocking the cyclical release of LH and FSH from the pituitary [Faloia *et al*, 1993]. They are available as nasal sprays (to be given 2 to 3 times a day), e.g. nafarelin and buserelin, subcutaneous injections (once daily), e.g. buserelin and leuprolide, intramuscular depot injection (to be given monthly), e.g. triptorelin and monthly subcutaneous implant (to be given monthly), e.g. leuprolin, Goserelin. Though GnRH analogues are very effective in suppressing ovarian androgen secretion, their use is limited by their high cost and menopausal symptoms including bone loss, on long term use. It does not incur contraception, hence nonhormonal contraception should be used simultaneously as pregnancy is contraindicated. Lactation, abnormal vaginal bleeding are other contraindications [Faloia *et al*, 1993].

2. Suppressor of Adrenal Androgen Secretion

Glucocorticoid: Glucocorticoids in low doses can suppress the adrenal production of androgens. They are indicated in patients who have an elevated level of DHEAS associated with an 11- or 21-hydroxylase deficiency. Low dose prednisolone (2.5 to 5 mg) or dexamethasone 0.25–0.75 mg night time dose, suppress adrenal androgen production [Pochi PE, 1982; Lucky A, 1995]. As this therapy has to be continued till the DHEAS is suppressed, which may take 3–6 months, it is better to use prednisolone than dexamethasone. Adrenal suppression is a possible side effect, for which ACTH stimulation test should be done 2–3 months after initiation of therapy. Glucocorticoids may also be used in acute flare or in very severe acne for a few weeks [Gollnick *et al*, 2003].

3. *Androgen Receptor Blockers*

a. *Spironalactone*: It is an androgen receptor blocker and an inhibitor of 5α *reductase* and an aldosterone antagonist. It has not formally been approved by FDA for acne, but it is often successfully used by dermatologists to treat hormone related acne, therapy resistant acne. It is administered in doses of 25 to 100 mg twice daily (e.g. aldactone). Side effects are dose dependent and include hyperkalemia, hypotension, irregular menstruation, headache, fatigue, breast tenderness, decreased libido, etc. Because pregnancy is an absolute contraindication as it can cause hypospadias and feminization of male fetus, its use with OCs is recommended. Response in acne can take as long as 3 months [Goodfellow *et al*, 1984].

b. *Flutamide*: Is an androgen receptor blocker. It has been used in doses of 250 mg twice a day in combination with oral contraceptives for the treatment of acne. Fatal hepatitis is a serious side effect and warrants monitoring of liver function test [Wysowski *et al*, 1993]. And in view of feminization of male fetus, pregnancy is contraindicated during therapy, hence concomitant OCs use is beneficial [Gollnick *et al*, 2003]. But use of flutamide is limited by its side effect profile.

c. *Cyproterone acetate*: Already discussed.

4. *5α Reductase Inhibitor*

Finasteride 5 mg/day is used by some dermatologists for hormone related acne. But more studies are needed to validate its use in acne. And concomitant OCs use is recommended with this drug [Kohler C *et al*, 2007].

5. *Insulin Sensitizer*

Metformin is used, especially in acne in association with PCOS, HAIR-AN syndrome, obese patients, or biochemical evidence of hyperinsulinemia. It is usually given in a dose of 500 mg OD to BD doses to up to 2000 mg/day. Most side effects are dose dependent and they are nausea, vomiting and lactic acidosis [Kazerooni T, *et al*, 2003]. Pioglitazone and rosiglitazone, also can be used for similar purpose[Costello M *et al*, 2007]. These insulin sensitizers may be used in combination with OCs or flutamide [Ibáñez L *et al*, 2006].

6. *Isotretinoin*

A recent study compared isotretinoin with conventional anti-androgens and found that there were no significant differences between using isotretinoin and cyproterone compounds in the treatment of acne in patients with SAHA syndrome or triad of cutaneous hyperandrogenism. This probably means, that in case of severe acne with features of hyperandrogenism, hormonal therapy can be initiated and used in combination with isotretinoin, if so indicated, to ensure a fast result.

Faghihi G, Jamshidi K, Tajmirriahi N, Abtahi-Naeini B, Nilforoshzadeh M, Radan M, Hosseini SM. The efficacy of oral isotretinoin versus cyproterone compound in female patients with acne and the triad of cutaneous hyperandrogenism: A randomized clinical trial. Adv Biomed Res. 2014 Dec 31;3:262.

REFERENCES

1. Cunliffe *et al*. Acne: Diagnosis and management. London: Martin Dunitz; 2001; p. 49–103.

2. Bhambri *et al*. Pathogenesis of acne vulgaris: recent adv, 2009.

3. Thiboutot. New treatments and therapeutic strategies for acne. Arch Fam Med 2000; 9:179–87ances. J Drugs Dermatol 2009; 8:615–8.

4. Simpson *et al*. Disorders of the sebaceous glands. In: Burns T, Breathnach S, Cox N, Griffiths C, editors. Rook's Textbook of Dermatology. 7 th ed. Blackwell Science; 2004. p. 43.1–43.75.

5. Harper JC. Antiandrogen therapy for skin disease and hair disease. Dermatol Clin 2006; 24:137–43.

6. George R, Clarke S, Thiboutot D. Hormonal therapy for acne. Semin Cutan Med Surg 2008; 27:188–96.

7. Goulden *et al*. Post-adolescent acne: a review of clinical features. The British Journal of Dermatology 1997; 136:66–70.

8. Gollnick *et al*. Management of acne: A report from a global alliance to improve outcomes in acne. J Am Acad Dermatol 2003; 49:S1–38.

9. Hormone therapy for acne Journal of the American Academy of Dermatology, Volume 62, Issue 3, pp 486–488 Jacqueline M. Junkins-Hopkins.

10. Pochi, PE: Hormones and acne. Semin Dermatol 1982 1:265.

11. Pochi PE. The pathogenesis and treatment of acne. Ann Rev Med 1990; 41:187–98.

12. Klingman *et al*. An investigation of the biology of the human sebaceous gland. J Invest Dermatol. 1958; 30:99–125.

13. Pochi *et al*. Sebaceous gland suppression with ethinyl oestradiol and diethyl stilboestrol. Arch Dermatol. 1973; 108:210-1.

14. Ehrmann *et al.* Endocrin Rev 1995; 16:322–53.

15. Chen *et al.* Cutaneous androgen metabolism: basic research and clinical perspective. J Invest Dermatol. 2002; 119:992–1007.

16. Schmidt *et al.* Hyperprolactinemia and hypophyseal hypothyroidism as cofactors in hirsutism and androgen-induced alopecia in women. Hautarzt 1991; 42:168–72.

17. Beylot *et al.* Oral Contraceptives and cyproterone acetate in female acne treatment. Dermatology 1998; 196:148–52.

18. Hormone therapy for acne Journal of the American Academy of Dermatology, Volume 62, Issue 3, 2010;pp 486-488 Jacqueline M. Junkins-Hopkins.

19. Lin-Su *et al.* Congenital adrenal hyperplasia in adolescents: Diagnosis and management. Ann N Y Acad Sci 2008; 1135:95–8.

20. Eric *et al.* Ovarian hormones and andrenal androgens during a women's life span. J Am Acad Dermatol 2001; 45:S105–15.

21. Chang *et al.* Diagnosis of polycystic ovary syndrome. Endocrinol Metab Clin North Am. 1999; 28:397–408.

22. Schmidt *et al.* Hyperprolactinemia and hypophyseal hypothyroidism as cofactors in hirsutism and androgen-induced alopecia in women. Hautarzt 1991; 42:168–72.

23. Ehrmann *et al.* Endocrin Rev 1995; 16:322–53.

24. Thiboutot D. Endocrinilogical evaluation and hormonal therapy for difficult acne. J Eur Acad Dermatol Venereol 2001; 15:57–61.

25. Arowojolu *et al.* Combined oral contraceptive pills for treatment of acne. Cochrane Database Syst Rev 2009; 3:CD004425.

26. Lucky *et al.* Effectiveness of norgestimate and ethinyl estradiol in treating moderate acne vulgaris. J Am Acad Dermatol 1997; 37:746–54.

27. Rothman *et al.* Acne vulgaris. Adv Dermatol 1993; 8:347–74; discussion, 375.

28. Harper JC. Should dermatologists prescribe hormonal contraceptives for acne? Dermatol Ther 2009; 22:452–7.

29. Murphy *et al.* The effect of tetracycline on levels of oral contraceptives. Am J Obstet Gynecol 1991; 164:28–33.

30. Haroun M. Hormonal therapy of acne. J Cutan Med Surg 2004; 8(Suppl 4):6–10.

31. Van Wayjen *et al.* Experience in the long-term treatment of patients with hirsutism and/or acne with cyproterone acetate-containing preparations: efficacy, metabolic, and endocrine effects. Exp Clin Endocrinol Diabetes 1995; 103:241–51.

32. Gollnick *et al*. Efficacité de l'acé tate de cyprotéone oral associe á l'é thinylestradiol dans le traitement de l'acne´ tardive de type facial. Ann Endocrinol 1999; 60:157–66.

33. Hammerstein *et al*. Use of cyproterone acetate (CPA) in the treatment of acne, hirsutism, and virilism. J Steroid Biochem 1975; 6:827–36.

34. Faloia *et al*. Treatment with a gonadotropin-releasing hormone agonist in acne or idiopathic hirsutism. J Endocrinol Invest 1993; 16:675.

35. Lucky A. Hormonal correlates of acne and hirsutism. Am J Med 1995; 98:89S–94S.

36. Goodfellow *et al*. Oral spiranolactone improves acne vulgaris and reduces sebum secretion. Br J Dermatol 1984; 111:209–14.

37. Wysowski *et al*. Fatal and nonfatal hepatotoxicity associated with flutamide. Ann Intern Med 1993; 118:860–4.

38. Kohler C *et al*. Effect of finasteride 5 mg (Proscar) on acne and alopecia in female patients with normal serum levels of free testosterone. Gynecol Endocrinol. 2007; 23:142–5.

39. Kazerooni T, *et al*. Effects of metformin therapy on hyperandrogenism in women with polycystic ovarian syndrome Gynecol Endocrinol. 2003; 17:51–6.

40. Costello M *et al*. Cochrane Database System rev. 2007; 1:CD005552.

41. Ibáñez L *et al*. Low-dose flutamide-metformin therapy for hyper-insulinemic hyperandrogenism in non-obese adolescents and women. Hum Reprod Update. 2006; 12:243–52.

Index